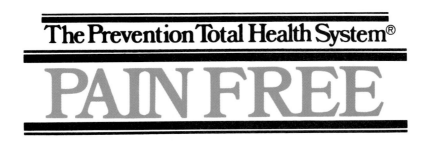

The Prevention Total Health System®

PAIN FREE

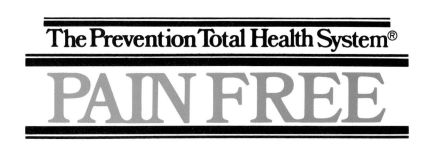

The Prevention Total Health System®

PAIN FREE

by the Editors of
Prevention® Magazine

 Rodale Press, Emmaus, Pennsylvania

Printed in the United States of America

Library of Congress Cataloging in Publication Data

Main entry under title:

Pain free.

(The Prevention total health system)
On t.p. the registered trademark symbol "R" is superscript following "Prevention" in the statement of responsibility and "system" in the series statement.
Includes index.
1. Pain—Treatment. 2. Analgesia.
I. Prevention (Emmaus, Pa.) II. Series. [DNLM:
1. Pain—prevention & control—popular works.
WL 704 P1455]
RB127.P33225   1986   616'.0472   85-28264

ISBN 0-87857-555-3   hardcover
     8   10   9   hardcover

NOTICE

The Prevention Total Health System®
Series Editors: William Gottlieb, Mark Bricklin
Supervising Editor: Carol Keough
Pain Free Editor: Stephen Williams
Writers: Stephen Williams (Chapters 1, 11); Dary Matera (Chapters 2, 6); Gerry Hunt (Chapters 3, 9); Mike McGrath (Chapters 4, 7); Ellen Michaud (Chapter 5); Gretchen Reynolds (Chapter 8) with Camille Cusumano and Jane Allison; Nona Cleland, Ellen Michaud (Chapter 10); Dary Matera, Sharon Faelten (Chapter 12).
Research Chief: Carol Baldwin
Associate Research Chief, Prevention Health Books: Susan Nastasee
Assistant Research Chief, Prevention Health Books: Holly Clemson
Researchers: Sue Ann Alleger, Jill Jurgensen, Sally Novack Lynda Pollack, Carole Rapp, Martin Wood
Copy Editor: Jane Sherman
Editorial Consultant: Carol A. Warfield, M.D.
Series Art Director: Jane C. Knutila
Designers: Lynn Foulk, Alison Lee
Project Assistants: Lisa Gatti, Margot J. Weissman
Illustrators: Bascove, Susan Blubaugh, Mellisa Edmonds, Susan Gray, Elwood Smith, Wendy Wray
Director of Photography: T. L. Gettings
Photo Editor: Margaret Skrovanek
Staff Photographers: Angelo M. Caggiano, Carl Doney, Donna Hornberger, Alison Miksch, Margaret Skrovanek
Photographic Stylists: Renee Keith, Debra Minotti
Photo Researcher: Donna Lewis
Production Manager: Jacob V. Lichty
Senior Production Coordinator: Barbara A. Herman
Production Coordinator: Eileen F. Bauder
Composite Typesetter: Brenda J. Kline
Production Assistant: Barbara Sellers
Office Personnel: Susan K. Lagler, Roberta Mulliner, Janet Schuler

Rodale Books, Inc.
Publisher: Thomas Woll
Senior Managing Editor: William H. Hylton
Assistant Managing Editor: Ann Snyder
Art Director: Jerry O'Brien
Director of Marketing: Pat Corpora
Director of Book Production, Trade Sales and Subsidiary Rights: Ellen J. Greene

Rodale Press, Inc.
Chairman of the Board: Robert Rodale
President: Robert Teufel
Executive Vice President: Marshall Ackerman
Group Vice Presidents: Sanford Beldon
                      Mark Bricklin
Senior Vice President: John Haberern
Vice Presidents: John Griffin
              James C. McCullagh
              David Widenmyer
Secretary: Anna Rodale

Contents

Successful Ways to Ease Pain

Learning to relieve pain must be the most gratifying health lesson
of them all.

Some people worry about their cholesterol count or their weight.
But what do these mere numbers mean compared to the electric sizzle of
sciatica or the brain-mashing hammer of migraine?

It's no good to be told that pain won't kill you when you already feel
you're in hell. Something has got to be done, and that's what this book
is all about.

Luckily, there's been a lot of good research into pain control in
recent years, so there are lots of valuable lessons to be learned. Clinics
devoted to pain relief have been opened by major health organizations,
and we have talked with experts at many of them in preparing this
volume of The Prevention Total Health System.® Their advice is
practical, not just theoretical, and based on actual treatments of many
patients. This is the kind of information we most like to present—the
kind that can make a big difference in how you feel.

What's perhaps most surprising about the new approach to pain
relief is that drugs play only a minor role. Too many drugs, doctors have
learned, are addictive. And often their effect seems to diminish rapidly
with continued use. That's a dangerous combination, leading to abuse,
dependency and a host of side effects.

The new emphasis is on natural healing—what *you* can do for
yourself, through lifestyle changes, attitude, psychological techniques,
exercise, physical therapy, even nutrition.

They're all here, and any one of them may be the right technique,
the successful technique, for you. And you needn't be living in agony to
benefit. Do you have chronic, low-grade back pain? Tennis elbow?
Muscle pain? Knee pain? Cramps? Occasional tension headaches? At
one time or another, I've had all of them! So working on *Pain Free* has
been a most valuable experience for me. I think reading it will benefit
you, too.

Executive Editor, **Prevention**® Magazine

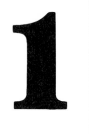

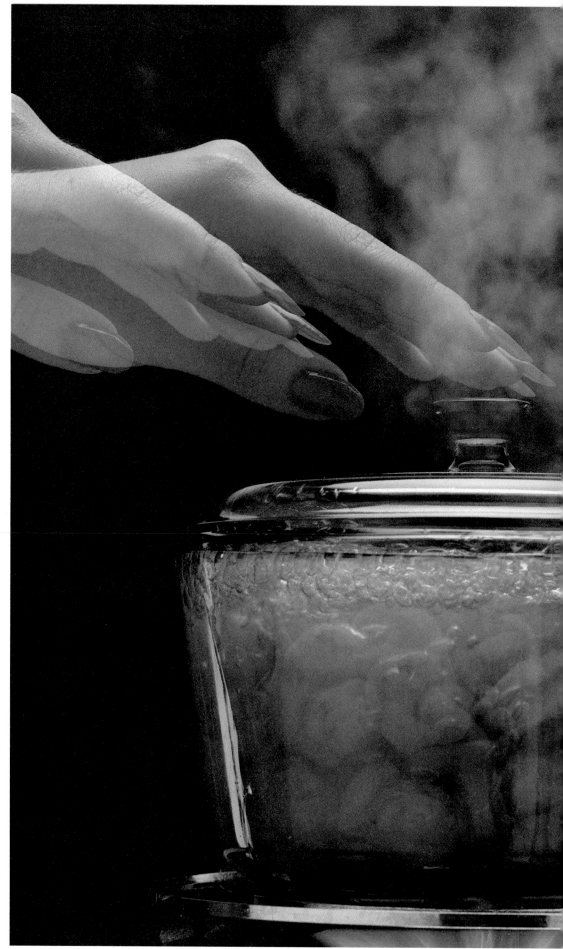

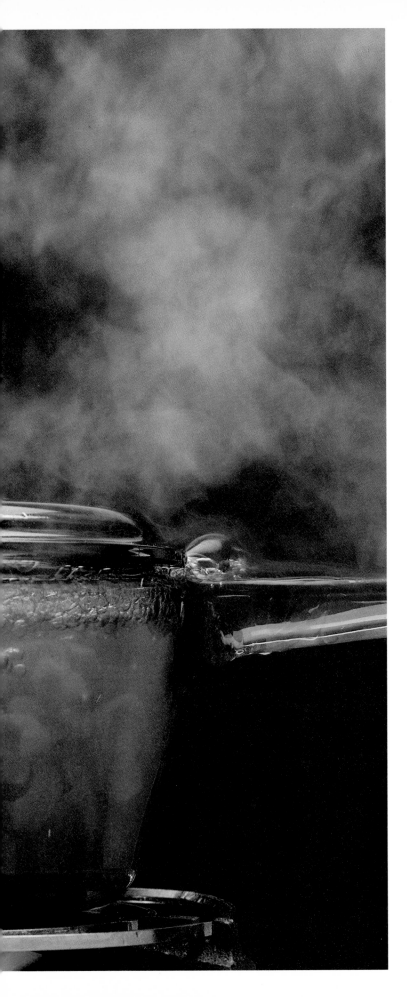

The Reason for Pain

Whether debilitating or just
irritating, pain serves
a vital purpose.

A sign hanging over a shop entrance in New
York City's Greenwich Village offers a kinky
choice: Ears Pierced, with or without Pain.
Not too many people are likely to stroll in and
ask for a pierced ear or two "with the pain, please."
No one needs to shop for pain, because there's
plenty to be had just for the taking. There's the
short-term, acute pain of cuts, sprains and occasional headaches, and the long-term, chronic pain
of rheumatoid arthritis, bone disease and slow-to-
heal injuries. There is slicing pain, burning pain,
scratching pain, stabbing pain—all in all, just too
much pain. And no matter what the type, most
people would be happy to give theirs away.

But they can't. Or more precisely, they and
their doctors don't always know how to. And
so they continue to suffer—but not alone. The
ranks of people with chronic pain are growing so
fast that one eminent pain researcher has suggested that "we may be living in an epidemic of
chronic pain."

In fact, pain is the most prevalent symptom
that sends people in search of health care. One
doctor, quoted in a national news weekly, estimates that $70 billion is spent each year in lost
workdays and medical bills by people suffering
from and trying to conquer chronic pain.

Does anyone find relief?

Yes. Though the large number of doctor visits
we make wouldn't suggest so, many people do find
ways to ease their pain. You can, too. This book
will tell you how.

It's good news for the millions of people who
want relief from a host of minor pains, as well as
crippling arthritis pain, disabling back pain,
excruciating migraine headaches and the savage
grip of other painful illnesses like sciatica
and gout.

Of course, you are probably already blessed

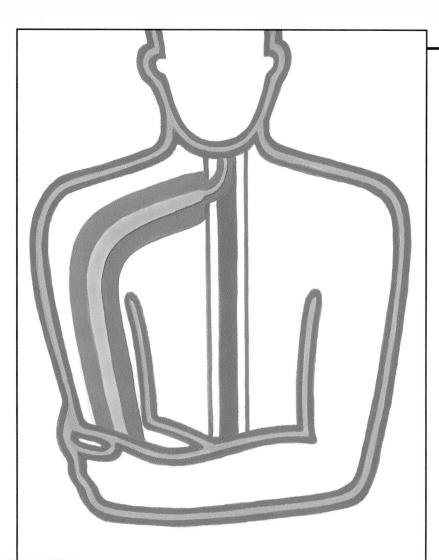

Closing the Gate of Pain

When your smack your elbow, you rub it to ease the pain, right? Each time you do that you're putting the gate-control theory of pain to practical use. Much of modern pain control is based on this theory. It says that injury sends impulses along three kinds of nerve fibers. C fibers, the thinnest and most prevalent, transmit pain impulses. A-Beta fibers, thicker and faster acting, carry painless sensations of touch and pressure. A-Delta fibers also carry pain, particularly that of a sudden injury.

When triggered by an injury to your elbow, all three nerves, but especially the A-Delta fibers, send impulses along your arm to the spine, where they come together and pass through a "gate" before going to the brain and making you wince with pain. But as you rub the elbow for relief, you stimulate A-Beta fibers. These nonpain impulses rush toward the brain, creating a logjam when they meet the other nerve impulses at the gate. The gate blocks almost all the impulses, reducing the pain you feel.

one useful bit of knowledge about how to cope with pain. This widely used technique for controlling acute pain doesn't even need a doctor's prescription: A stiff upper lip. Sooner rather than later, acute pain is going to pass. The only problem is that the wait hurts.

But there are other, less heroic and more satisfying health tips you can learn to speed the relief of acute pain, like the right way to apply cold or heat to an injury and how to find the right over-the-counter drug in the most effective dose.

Chronic pain is another matter, however, and can't be so easily overcome. By definition, it is a brawny contender. But it's not an unbeatable one.

The key to relief from chronic pain is understanding the many options that are available. You don't bash this type of pain, you outwit it. And while there often is no quick cure, different combinations of exercise, drugs, biofeedback, electrical stimulation and other therapies can give you control over your pain. You just have to know what's available and how to use it.

The first step is to learn exactly what you're dealing with.

WHAT IS PAIN?

Pain is what makes you scream, swear and dance around. When you casually lean against the hot metal burner of the stove while explaining the secret of your just-sauteed feast to an inquisitive guest, pain makes you pull away fast. You learn early that pain isn't something you want to feel, and this knowledge makes you unconsciously cautious about many things, like fires, rusty nails and falls from trees. And when you do injure yourself, pain keeps you from aggravating the injury.

In this sense, pain is good. It hurts but it also protects you and forces you to take care of yourself. Without it your life would be miserable—and probably short.

PULSATIONS OF PAIN

The best-understood type of pain is the kind that accompanies an injury,

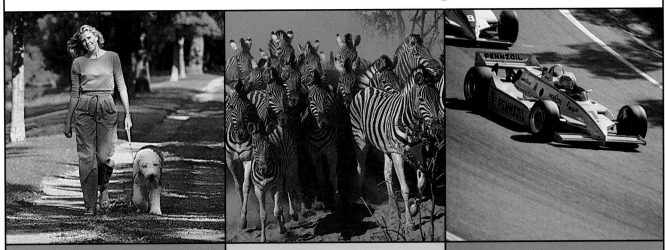

Race of the Pain Messengers

C Fibers

Pain signals amble along tiny C fibers at less than 3 miles per hour. Slow but abundant, they cause a second, aching type of pain.

A-Delta Fibers

Pain signals pulse along some of the smaller A-Delta fibers at a brisk 40 miles per hour. When triggered, they create some of the first, sharp pains of an injury.

A-Beta Fibers

Touch and pressure sensations zoom along large A-Beta fibers at speeds of 180 to 200 miles per hour. They can close the "gate" and block the pain signals.

like a bruised rib or a scraped knee. This type of pain makes sense to everyone: It is a warning signal, reminding you that part of the body is damaged.

When you hurt yourself, nerves in the skin and tissue convey small electric currents from the injury to your brain. Different nerves, or pain receptors, send different messages. There are receptors that detect damage such as crushing and tearing, others that detect heat and cold, and still others that respond to all types of sensations. They all work together to tell your brain what is happening to your body, so you can decode just what the problem is—whether it is a shard of glass piercing your foot or a snake biting it.

Most of these receptors are in your skin, though some are deep in your body. What you feel depends on the type of receptors that are near the injury. There are almost no crush-

ing, burning or cutting receptors in the intestines, for instance, so they could be cut, crushed or burned without your feeling much pain. But the intestines do have plenty of receptors—some people would say too many—that sense when they are bloated with gas or wracked with spasms.

Muscles have different pain receptors that feel other kinds of pain. Chemical toxins produced by the body during any kind of exertion, including walking up the stairs or running, can cause pain even when there is no apparent injury, such as a sprain.

In addition to those created by exertion, the body also releases other chemicals that cause pain. The monthly torment of menstrual cramps, for example, is due to chemicals called prostaglandins, which cause the muscles of the uterus to contract. Uterine contractions are necessary during childbirth, but otherwise the pain seems to be just needless suffering.

Yet prostaglandins do serve a useful purpose. These are some of the same chemicals that sensitize the pain receptors around an injury, reminding you to favor it by limping or cradling the area. And they trigger the swelling that acts as a sort of splint to further protect the area.

Still other pain-producing body chemicals are called kinins. Whenever there is inflammation, as in arthritis, kinins are released, stimulating the receptors in the area and causing great pain. And the combined effect of the kinins and the prostaglandins that always hang around when there is inflammation means double trouble. Their vicious interaction with the pain receptors is partly responsible for the kind of painful inflammation that just seems to get worse and worse, as is the case with much arthritis.

NAVIGATING THE PAIN PATHWAYS

Whatever the cause of your pain, the electrical impulses that carry it travel through your body on distinct pathways, moving through the tissue from nerve fiber to nerve fiber to the spinal cord and the "gate," before finally reaching the brain. (See "Closing the Gate of Pain" on page 2.)

Once the impulses hit the brain, you feel pain. Just what kind of pain depends on which nerve fibers deliver the message. (See "Race of the Pain Messengers" on page 3.)

Immediately after an injury, you feel "first pain." It is usually the most excruciating and is the pain you feel when you break a bone or crack a tooth. These first pain signals are delivered quickly along the nervous system's A-Delta fibers.

The fast messages of these fibers are what signal you to pull away from pain—if possible—seemingly before you feel it. If you spill steaming coffee onto your hand, for instance, you will probably drop the cup on the floor before you even realize that you've been burned. This reflexive response happens when the signals sent over A-Delta fibers reach receptors in the spinal cord, which immediately tell the muscles in your body to get your hand away from the pain—they don't give you time to think about how the coffee will stain the carpet when you drop the cup. The whole sequence happens as the signals travel through your body.

Then, a little while after the A-Delta fibers do their job, most people feel a dull ache. It's not as sharp as the initial stabbing pain, but it can be more bothersome. This second type of pain is delivered mainly by the C fibers, and it can last a long time.

"C" doesn't stand for chronic—but it could. Also for constant and crippling (at least emotionally). That's the nature of pain that doesn't go away: You feel the pain, yet you also anticipate that it will be with you in an hour, in a year, forever. Many people with chronic pain lead lives that are devoted to thinking about a future not of days of work followed by evenings of relaxation, but of excruciating minute upon minute of pain, until the minutes add up to a tortured life.

Often this pain is due to a physical cause, such as arthritis or irritable bowel syndrome. But sometimes there is no apparent cause and the pain is inexplicable, though still very real.

Pain like this can be the most frustrating of all, because there seems to be no cause and no cure, yet the pain exists. This type of pain almost makes pain with a traceable physical root seem like a blessing.

PAIN THAT IS A MYSTERY

"There isn't a distinct physical reason for every pain, and some can be very difficult to detect by the non-expert. But no matter wht the cause, the pain hurts," says Steven Brena, M.D., chairman of the Pain Control and Rehabilitation Institute of Georgia, Inc. "Someone who says they have pain is in pain." adds John Loeser, M.D., of the pain clinic at the University of Washington in Seattle.

In Los Angeles, a motorcycle cop visited doctors at a university pain clinic and complained of severe,

"Corinne Doe"
Insensitivity to Pain

Corinne stares at her twisted limb. At the ankle, her right foot buckles gruesomely inward where the broken bones failed to meet. Five scarred and ulcerated toes peer from behind the traction apparatus as the 11-year-old looks on, puzzled. She has spent much of her life in hospital beds, but there is one thing she has never understood. "They tell me it should hurt," she says, "but it doesn't. I don't know what pain feels like."

Corinne is a composite of several people, but the stories of others with the extremely rare disorder called congenital insensitivity to pain are remarkably similar. In every case, their nerves, reflexes and senses appear to be normal, but for reasons we don't understand, they cannot feel pain in any part of their bodies. As a result, from birth to adulthood, they unknowingly bruise and mutilate themselves because they never feel the warning signals of pain.

Corinne repeatedly injures her fingers and toes—so much that the tips actually wear away. While eating food, she scars the inside of her mouth and bites off the end of her tongue. She suffers recurrent skin, hand and foot infections, which often go unnoticed, and she once ruptured her eardrum without complaint.

Compounding these severe problems is the more visible damage Corinne has done to her bones and joints. By the time she was 9, she had fractured her left hip and broken her right leg twice. Her joints became swollen and deformed because she never shifted her weight when standing and didn't roll over in her sleep. Finally, she broke her right ankle in a fall, but ignored the fracture until it healed into a C-shaped curve, necessitating the traction device that hangs at the foot of her bed.

The misshapen ankle reminds Corinne of her doctor's earlier advice. "We hope she'll learn to limit her behavior as she matures," he had explained to her mother. "She'll have to inspect her shoes daily for nails or stones and continually monitor her body for signs of other injury. Unfortunately, she also cannot feel internal pain, so it's possible she could rupture her appendix or suffer a heart attack without realizing it."

Falling back on her pillow, Corinne sighs. Suddenly wise beyond her years, she remembers the doctor's final words. "Corinne's handicap is severe," he had stressed. "Pain is one of the body's most important signals. Without it, it's impossible to lead a normal life."

repeated headaches. The doctors were puzzled by this tall, tough, beefy cop complaining of chronic pain with no apparent cause. Following tests that ruled out disease or other organic causes, the doctors finally concluded that his pain was an expression of the stress he experienced as a result of being a cop. People were rude to him all the time, his job was violent and he felt constantly exposed to danger on his motorcycle. Somehow the pain was a response to his environment. He needed to learn ways to cope with his stress.

A Bangor, Maine, mother flew her daughter all the way to the pain clinic at the University of Washington in Seattle in a desperate attempt to get the girl the best treatment possible for her pain. She was 21 years old and had suffered severe shoulder and abdominal pain since she was 17. A series of doctors up and down the East Coast had tried almost every medical treatment available in an attempt to banish her pain, including TENS, bone scans, biofeedback and surgery—all to no avail.

When the Seattle doctors gathered in conference to discuss the case, the examining doctor said he could find no physical cause for her pain, but he believed that her suffering was very real. Then the psychologist spoke up. His interview with the woman had convinced him that her pain had an emotional basis, though the specific causes couldn't be pinpointed. "She's a bundle of contradictions," he said. "She prides herself on being tough, but she's really weak and always in pain; she has created a grand myth that she's had to make it through life on her own, even though her mother has been with her at every turn to provide a nice home and food on the table; she'll say at one point that she'll kill herself unless she finds relief from her pain soon, then turns around and admits that she really couldn't go through with suicide and never thought she could; she's fixated on finding the best treatment and the quickest cure, but she never stays with one doctor long enough to find relief. She is guarded, defensive and obsessed with her body and her pain," concluded the psychologist.

After a discussion of the possible treatments, the doctors decided to accept the young woman for treatment. Their job: to help her cut her apron strings from her mother; to get her off drugs; to teach her to focus on things other than her body and her pain; and to help her reduce her stress levels.

At the Emory University Pain Control Center, a wiry, gray-haired woman with a face that somehow showed friendliness and hope despite lines of misery told her doctors that she hadn't sat down for more than a minute or two in two years. She had seen countless doctors and none could tell her what was wrong. But her pain was real. It made her clutch a pillow to protect her arm and lean against another pillow propped between her and the cement-block wall. As she spoke, her pain caused her to shift from leg to leg. The doctors at the clinic were faced with the problem of developing a way to teach her to cope with her pain. Of course, these people who suffer from mysterious pain are only a few of the many whose puzzling conditions challenge the skills of those who staff pain clinics.

But the mystery of pain is not only in pain without apparent cause. Sometimes it's just the opposite; sometimes a person *should* be in pain but isn't. The following story is a good—if scary—example.

DR. LIVINGSTONE AND THE LION

David Livingstone, famous as the man Henry Stanley combed Africa in search of, was on a low grassy hill when he was attacked by a large lion. He describes the experience in his book, *Livingstone's Africa*, published in 1872:

"I heard a shout. Staring and looking half round, I saw the lion just in the act of springing upon me. I was on a little height; he caught my shoulder as he sprang and we both came to the ground below together. Growling horribly close to my ear, he shook me as a terrier does a rat. The shock produced a stupor similar to that which seems to be felt by a mouse after the first shake of a cat. It caused a sort of dreaminess in which there was no sense of pain nor feeling of terror, though (I was) quite conscious of all that was happening. It was like what patients partially under the influence of chloroform describe, who see all the operation but feel not the knife. This singular condition was not the result of any mental process. The shake annihilated fear, and allowed no sense of horror in looking round at the beast. The peculiar state is probably produced in all animals killed by carnivora; and if so, is a merciful provision by our benevolent Creator for lessening the pain of death."

Today people rarely face the beasts of the jungle. Yet many— particularly those with chronic pain— would welcome such a "merciful provision" to end their suffering. Instead, the key to their relief is often not to end the pain outright but to learn how to not feel it, to not let it be part of their lives.

That's not impossible, says Dr. Sampson Lipton, retired director of the Centre for Pain Relief at Walton Hospital in Liverpool, England, because the body already has a built-in mechanism that can help screen out some types of pain. Your nervous system, he explains, is continually receiving a vast amount of information from your skin, muscles, eyes, ears, toes, internal organs and more. "If all this information were allowed to go straight into your conscious brain, you would be completely overwhelmed by it," he writes in *Conquering Pain.* "Since much of this information is not important, there is no point in a great deal of it reaching conscious level and, in fact, most of it does not." This process of modulation is what can keep some pain from registering. "You can distract your conscious mind from recognizing pain," says Dr. Lipton.

Making chronic pain "not important" by emphasizing the importance of other areas in your life—work, family, recreation—can help stop pain.

PAIN BY ANY OTHER NAME HURTS LESS

Some of the differences in pain thresholds among different people can be explained by how they express their pain. As Dr. Loeser says, people are feeling just as much pain as they *say* they feel.

Scientists W. Crawford Clark, Ph.D., of Columbia University in New York City, and Susanne Bennett Clark, Ph.D., of Boston University, were drawn all the way to the high Himalayan Mountains to find out why some people seem to feel less pain than others. They compared the pain thresholds of Nepalese mountain porters, accustomed to carrying heavy packs at high altitudes in freezing cold while wearing only light clothing, with those of Westerners who, though familiar with the minor hardships of camping at lower altitudes, were used to a more plush lifestyle.

When tested with electrically

PHANTOM
Pain from Nowhere

The patient's index finger just kept on aching— even though he had lost it in an industrial accident months earlier. He thought he was crazy until doctors told him that many amputees suffer from phantom limb pain—excruciating pains in legs, arms and even breasts that have been surgically removed.

Fortunately, doctors know that phantom pain isn't imagined. "There's a very real cause for it," says Richard Sherman, Ph.D., a psychophysiologist at the Army Medical Center in Fort Gordon, Georgia. Pain signals from distant nerves normally go to corresponding places in the brain's own map of the body, he explains. This mental diagram dictates where pain will be felt, but for unknown reasons it sometimes short-circuits, resulting in phantom pain. Even if a leg has been amputated, changes in temperature, blood flow and muscle tension or stimulation of the severed nerve will still send signals to the brain's map, leading it to think the leg is still there. Relaxation techniques and electrical stimulation often help relieve the pain, while "wiggling" the phantom limb, imagining it's being heated, or massaging the stump to promote blood flow also give relief.

induced pain, the Nepalese porters showed much higher pain thresholds than the Westerners. And the difference wasn't in how much pain they felt but in how it affected them. The Nepalese were much more tolerant of pain. According to the scientists, "The high pain threshold of the Nepalese is due to their stoicism, probably induced by their harsh living conditions, and perhaps in part by other ethnocultural factors such as religion."

Differences in pain tolerance can also be seen in the Plains Indians, who once performed a difficult ceremonial Sun Dance in which they pierced the skin of their chests with skewers attached to ropes. The ropes were pulled up, causing what would be, for those in many cultures, excruciating pain. For the Plains Indians, the pain was accepted as being a part of their rite of passage.

Another factor that affects pain is mood. As one patient at the Johns Hopkins Pain Treatment Center in Baltimore told his doctor, "When I don't feel pain, I don't feel depressed, and when I don't feel depressed, I don't feel pain. It's as simple as that." In fact, depression and chronic pain often go hand in hand. Anxiety and agitation also boost the perception of pain.

IF YOU BELIEVE IT HURTS, IT HURTS

Finally, your belief system can affect your perception of pain. A good example of this—albeit a fantastic one—occurs among members of the cult of *obeah*, in the backwaters of Louisiana. For them pain is something that can be visited on a person in the form of a curse. To cause the pain, according to this system, you need a Bible and a voodoo doll. First you read Psalm 109, repeating the victim's name at the end of each verse until you reach verse 20. From then on you just read the psalm alone. Then you stick a black-headed pin into the part of the doll where you want the victim to feel pain.

A person who thinks he's under this spell may actually feel pain, though nonbelievers might dismiss it as hogwash. And aspirin and biofeedback won't relieve it. The only way the pained believer can relieve his misery is by carrying two bags of coltsfoot, yellow dock, sassafrass, comfrey, hyssop and olive oil wrapped in green cloth and tied with red string, then wrapped in red cloth.

In other words, says Dr. Brena, "Pain is what the person feeling it says it is. Pain can be many things. It can be any one, any combination, or *all* of the following: a distressing, unpleasant experience; a learned behavior; a symptom of a disease; or even an expression of psychosocial malaise." And whatever the reason for their pain, everyone wants a cure.

THE CURE FOR PAIN

As you can see, pain can take many forms and have many causes. But what can be done about it?

How Pains Compare

Although pain is hard to gauge because everyone feels it differently, scientists using a test called the McGill questionnaire asked people to rate their pain at a point along a scale. As you can see, the result is a good argument for remembering to send flowers on Mother's Day.

Since time began, the quest for pain relief has sent humans searching for quick, lasting relief—for a magic cure. Painkilling drugs such as opium, cocaine, marijuana and mandrake root have been used for thousands of years. Impressively complicated machines to generate "painkilling" static electricity were widely used in the 18th century, and Rube Goldberg-like contraptions have been touted as pain relievers by opportunistic inventors ever since.

People in search of quick cures have had their bodies operated on, their bones reshaped, and their minds read. They've even traveled great distances to sit in abandoned radioactive mines in Montana—all in the quest for pain relief.

Many have found relief, but most have learned that "magic" cures don't last. What's needed are treatments that are medically sound, not ones that just sound medical.

And pain has to be kept in a realistic perspective. Chronic, hard-to-treat pain has to be viewed as some-

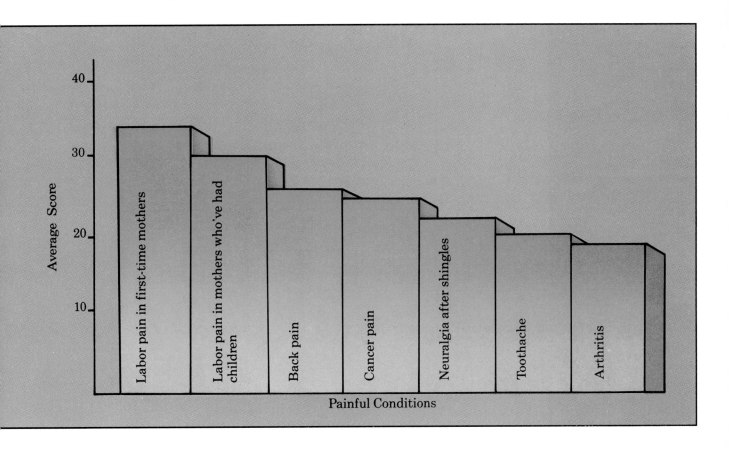

thing more than just an irritation or a symptom of simple injury. It can be caused by many things in the mind and the body, and it might take a broad treatment program to relieve it.

You have to be willing to learn about treatments like visual imagery, TENS, relaxation therapy and drug therapy, and then you have to work with your doctor to set up an effective treatment program. The information is available, but only you can put it to work.

"If you have a barking dog outside your window, but you are happy and busy, you'll ignore the dog," says Dr. Brena. "But if you aren't happy, and don't do anything about the dog, the dog will drive you crazy. That's the same with pain. If you always think about it and don't do anything about it, you will get depressed and the pain will win."

And proof that you can silence the barking dog is apparent in the different attitudes of the patients on their first day at Dr. Brena's clinic and in the final days before they leave. On their first day the patients get an introductory lecture in a pleasant room that seems far removed from the clinical setting one expects, but their faces are anything but relaxed or hopeful. Most look as though they came to the clinic because they couldn't think of any other option; as if they'd heard it all before but figured they might as well give it a try. Their faces register pain and disillusionment; some seem too weary to pay attention. But working and struggling to overcome their suffering pays off. In the final days of their several-week stay their faces are hopeful—and sometimes incredulous—because they've switched roles with their pain. They've become master of their bodies once again. And so can you.

"The attitude that works for people in pain should be that of a person who will earn a million dollars for doing something," Dr. Brena says.

Wouldn't being free of pain seem that valuable to you?

9

2

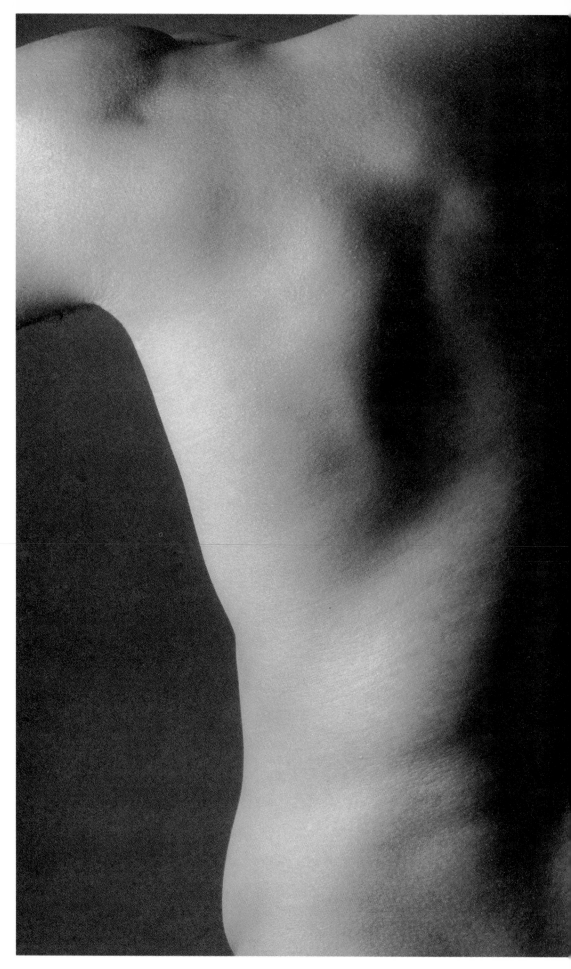

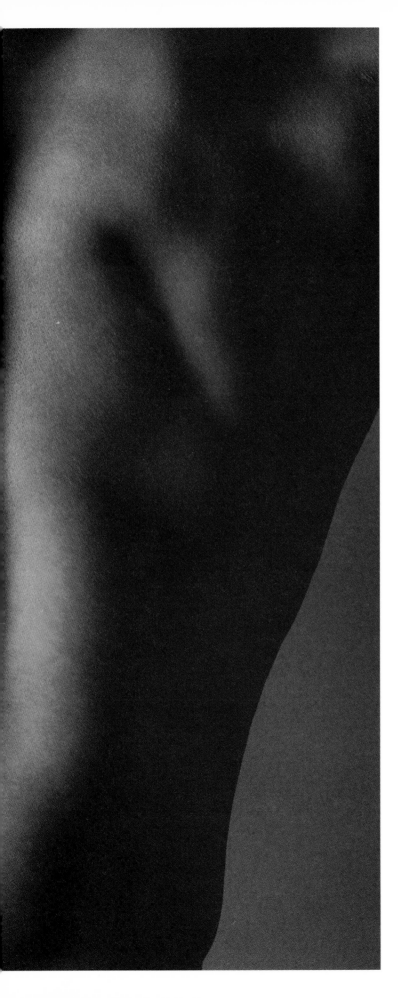

Beating Back and Neck Pain

Put that pain behind you
—for good—with stress relief,
proper lifting techniques and
easy exercise.

Easy to get, hard to cure. That's back and neck pain in a nutshell. These persistent and resistant problems have become a literal pain in the neck for doctors to treat. They've spawned a dizzying and often contradictory array of treatments. One prominent surgeon preaches "no pain, no gain," and puts his patients through exercises that hurt at first, but offer pain relief in the long run. Another doctor swears that the key is battling mental stress and tension. Others advocate manipulation, acupuncture, acupressure, dance —even the pretzel postures of yoga that seem like they'd kink your spine, not straighten it.

"There is probably no other medical condition which is treated in so many different ways and by such a variety of practitioners as back pain," admits John Sarno, M.D., author of the book *Mind over Back Pain.*

But that doesn't have to be a bad thing, says Nelson Hendler, M.D., a psychiatrist and pain expert at Johns Hopkins Hospital and the Mensana Clinic in Baltimore. The trick, he believes, is to *use* the many ways to treat—and cure—back pain, to not limit yourself to one method.

"If all you have is a hammer, everything begins to look like a nail," he says, criticizing the one-method approach. But the diagnosis and management of chronic pain demands knowledge of *many* fields, including basic biochemistry, pharmacology, neuroanatomy, orthopedics, neurosurgery, rheumatology, psychiatry, neurodiagnostic studies and even sociology and the law.

"Of course, this Superdoctor doesn't exist," Dr. Hendler admits. But you can create the next best thing: A treatment program that gives you the right combination of therapies to ease your pain.

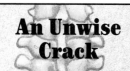

An Unwise Crack

"Don't go to the doctor," offers a confident friend. "Let me crack your back and you'll be as good as new." While your buddy may give you some relief, most doctors say you could be setting yourself up for serious injury.

"Cracking your back is monkey business," says C. James Greenwood, Jr., M.D., former chief of neuro-surgery and neurology at Baylor College of Medicine, Houston. "If you have a loose disk and ligaments, you can pop them in and out and there's a real potential for serious damage. Even if you avoid damage, you could actually make the problem worse because the object is to tighten the ligaments with exercise, not loosen them by cracking the back."

That's exactly what we do in this chapter. By gathering the latest techniques from the experts who have made victory over back and neck pain their life's work, we've created a practical version of that wondrous multidisciplinary Superdoc who can help free you from misery.

THE CAUSE OF BACK PAIN: IS IT MUSCLES OR BONES?

A great deal of the problem in painbusting the back lies in the multitude of causes that can produce the agony. The list itself is back-breaking. Physical strain, flat feet, bladder problems, trauma, tension, spasm, degenerative arthritis, mis-aligned muscles and bones, bad posture, soft beds, lousy chairs, high heels, overweight, a short leg, jogging, injured disks, spine curvatures, inflammation, pinched nerves and a host of other unpleasantries have all been blamed. In the past, doctors leaned toward skeletal and structural damage as the main culprit. Surgery was often performed and frequently didn't help. But today, progressive doctors believe that *muscular* problems cause 80 to 90 percent of all back pain.

"Many of the people I see have disk abnormalities and a variety of structural problems, but we almost always conclude that these are not causing the pain," says Dr. Sarno, a physiatrist (an M.D. who uses a variety of treatments, including heat, water and exercise, to fight chronic medical conditions) and professor of clinical rehabilitation medicine at New York University School of Medicine. "In fact," he points out, "it is unusual for anyone over 30 not to have some structural abnormalities—a piece of bone missing, transitional vertebrae, curvatures, bone spurs, early signs of arthritis, bulging or herniated disks, narrowing of disk space—the list goes on. Yet in my practice, only 2 percent have pain due to any of these." Then what does Dr. Sarno believe causes most pain? "Virtually every patient has tension myositis syndrome—muscle spasm and nerve pain caused by constricted blood vessels due to tension and stress," he states.

"The first technique in fighting back pain," he continues, "is to

accept tension and stress as a major cause. This will allow you to over-come the fear that the pain is coming from a major *physical* disorder. Since fear itself is extremely stressful, those who can eliminate it may, in some cases, find immediate relief. Without this first step, exercise, physical therapy and other techniques will have little value."

Dr. Sarno says that even the vast majority of backs that "go out" are the result of nothing more than painful but treatable muscle spasms caused by stress and tension.

For immediate relief, he suggests applying moist heat in the form of a hot bath or shower or a hot tub. He sometimes prescribes a painkiller for one or two days to get people through the acute phase.

GIVE YOUR BACK A LIFT

A lifetime of chronic back pain, fed by stress, tension and anxiety, can be ignited by a simple strain. Despite this, experts say we give our backs the Rodney Dangerfield treatment—no respect.

"America's lifting techniques are horrible," says Jack R. Tessman, Ph.D., a physics professor at Tufts University in Medford, Massachusetts, who advises doctors and industries on body mechanics. "There has been considerably more emphasis on exercise to cure the problem than on the appropriate ways to avoid the pain in the first place. The emphasis is wrong."

An example: You drop a quarter. What do you do? You bend forward at the waist and scoop it up. No wonder back pain strikes 90 percent of the population at some point! That's exactly what Dr. Tessman says you're *not* supposed to do. He feels the toe-touch pick-up maneuver (along with toe-touch exercises) "is exactly the type of motion that makes the back muscles work with great force, compressing the spine."

If the object is a box of books or a car tire, the strain can lead to lingering back pain. The proper way to lift something is to squat down, bending at the knees. If it's a large object, lift it slightly to the side. One arm should be outstretched, with the hand underneath the object; the

Specialists in Relief

When researchers went right to back pain sufferers and asked which type of health professional gave them the best relief, the answers were a surprise. Dava Sobel and Arthur C. Klein report in *Backache Relief* that sometimes those with the least specialized medical training—even those with no training—are the best at relieving back pain. Judge the responses for yourself.

Specialist	Number of specialists in this survey	Provided dramatic long-term help	Provided moderate long-term help	Provided temporary help	Ineffective	Made patient feel worse
Orthopedist (orthopedic surgeon)	429	13%	10%	9%	61%	7%
General Practitioner (GP, family practitioner, internist)	266	8%	12%	14%	54%	12%*
Osteopath (osteopathic physician, doctor of osteopathy)	71	7%	21%	15%	46%	11%
Neurosurgeon	53	13%	13%	8%	51%	15%
Neurologist	44	2%	2%	4%	76%	16%
Physiatrist (doctor of physical medicine, doctor of rehabilitative medicine, physiatrician)	30	33%	53%	0%	7%	7%
Acupuncturist	25	16%	20%	32%	28%	4%
Rheumatologist	15	7%	33%	20%	40%	0%
Chiropractor	422	14%	14%	28%	33%	11%
Physical Therapist (physiotherapist)	140	34%	31%	8%	17%	10%
Dance Instructor	10	50%	40%	0%	0%	10%

*This high figure is due primarily to adverse reactions from prescription drugs.

other hand should grip the side or top. For objects that can be picked up with one hand, Dr. Tessman suggests placing your free hand on a solid object for support.

"The best advice is to lift things behind you. People just aren't used to that. If it's a heavy object on the floor, raise it up one side at a time onto a low stool or something for elevation, then lift it behind you," advises Dr. Tessman, author of the book *My Back Doesn't Hurt Anymore*.

Here are some more tips from Dr. Tessman:

• Get out of bed by pushing yourself up and forward and swinging your legs around.

• Put on socks by bringing your feet up one at a time, not bending your body down, or lie back in bed and put them on.

• Do you have a child or a grandchild? Don't reach over the crib railing to pick up the child. That's a back killer. Remove or lower the railing and bend your knees to lift the toddler.

• "Lifting heavy bags out of grocery carts can be a real back buster," says Dr. Tessman. "I'm amazed people don't use more

Seeing through X Rays

If your back doctor relies heavily on X rays, he may be looking right through your problem. Some top physicians today feel that the structural wear and tear of the spine that shows up in X rays is normal and not necessarily the cause of your pain. In fact, some doctors say that even damage as obvious as a herniated disk doesn't cause pain. These doctors feel that up to 90 percent of back pain may be caused by muscular problems. And since muscles don't appear on X rays, doctors who flash photos and point out "defects" are usually off target. X rays do reveal breaks, cancer, tuberculosis and other severe ailments, but such problems account for only a small percentage of back pain. Once these diseases are ruled out, X rays have little value.

plastic bags with handles. Invest in ten of those and use them more than once. If you must use paper bags, have them packed lighter."

- When they spade or dig, gardeners should dig to their sides, as though they were rowing a boat, and throw the material behind them.

- Open windows by facing away and lifting up behind you.

- When carrying trunks, sofas or mattresses, lift from behind.

- Give your trash can the respect it deserves. Drag it behind you. Or better yet, put it on wheels or a hand truck.

- Suitcases should be placed slightly behind you when lifting them. If you can, carry one in each hand for balance. The best thing is to put them on wheels.

SITTING, SLEEPING AND STANDING

This may floor you—literally.

If you're looking for one quick cure for chronic back pain, your bed might be the place to start. Some people find relief by switching to a softer bed, like a water bed. Still others find that a harder bed does the trick. If you think you need a harder bed, you might want to go all the way and try sleeping on the floor. Surprisingly, this simple step may permanently end years of back agony. The reason? Soft, sagging mattresses cause pain in some people by forcing back muscles to work all night to align the spine. Eliminate the cause and you've defeated the problem.

Unfortunately, sleeping on the floor can be a chore. Stomach sleepers rarely endure hard surfaces because of discomfort to knees and elbows. Back sleepers might toss and turn over to less comfortable positions. Snugglers might find their mates aren't loyal, compassionate or passionate enough to join them. If you're having a hard time with the floor, see "The Right Bed for Your Back," on page 20, for help in putting a little backbone in your bed.

DON'T GIVE YOURSELF THE CHAIR

Second to beds as back pain villains are chairs. If your job has you planted in a chair, you have problems enough.

"Sitting is a stressful position," says David Lehrman, M.D., chief of orthopedic surgery and director of the St. Francis Hospital Spine Center and Back School in Miami Beach, Florida. "Anything that stresses the spine will give you trouble if you hold that position for any length of time," he explains.

Add to that the stress of working hunched over a typewriter, drawing table, computer or desk, and you have the potential for serious pain. The key here is the word *potential*, because relief can be as easy as buying a new chair, like one that has adjustments for both the height and back. And use the adjustments! Tighten the chair's back if the "give" is too generous. The seat should be fairly flat, sturdy, and easily adjustable to different positions. It should be high enough to let you comfortably place the soles of your shoes on the floor, while the seat depth should end 6 to 8 inches from the knee. (When you have no choice of what to sit in, like on an airplane, take along a cushion designed to support your lower back. Many stores and catalogs sell these.) You should generally avoid canvas chairs and backless stools, because both are notorious back beaters.

However, there is one exception: the Balans chair. This chair has been specifically designed to use slants and knee rests to ease back pain. It consists of a backless seat slanted slightly down toward two slanted knee cushions. The Balans chair can be purchased at many furniture stores and from some catalogs. Test one first to see if it will help you.

Whatever chair you choose, be certain that it is in harmony with your desk. Generally, your desk should be level with your elbows when you sit upright.

For those times when you're just standing around the water cooler, the key to avoiding pain is good posture. And the secret of good posture is

(continued on page 18)

Joan Throckmorton
New York, N.Y.
Back Pain

Fueled by energy, determination and enthusiasm, Joan Throckmorton decided to carve a niche for herself in New York's high-pressure publishing industry. Intrigued by direct mail marketing of books and magazines, she formed her own firm, Joan Throckmorton, Inc., in 1968. It was a success, and has rewarded the 54-year-old entrepreneur with independence, financial security, a sense of accomplishment and a bad back. Her quest for relief epitomizes the difficulty people often have trying to treat this bewildering ailment.

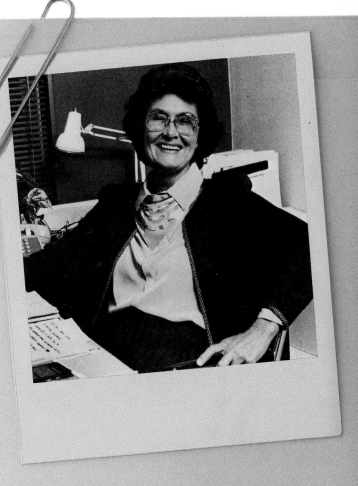

"It started out as minor, insignificant pain. It grew into a sciatic nerve problem that thrust pain down my right leg. When it first appeared, about 15 years ago, it would come and go. Then the last time it happened, last year, it wouldn't go away. It kept getting worse. There were sharp, shooting pains combined with a constant dull pain. I had a slight numbness in the toes, and extreme muscle contractions in the back and gluteal [buttocks] muscles.

"The cause? It depended on which doctor I saw. The first one, an arthritis specialist, told me it was arthritis. But after a long series of tests, he decided I was normal. He sent me to a neurologist who said I had deteriorated disks. He prescribed medicine and told me to immobilize myself and avoid walking.

"I went to a chiropractor about the same time. He said he could ease the pain with manipulation, stretching and traction stimulation exercises. He wanted me to come for therapy 2 or 3 times a week. At this point, I had spent a fortune for a lot of diagnosis and little relief.

"Finally, I went to Dr. John Sarno, at the New York University Medical Center.

He has a revolutionary new theory that most back pain is caused by stress. He said that the last thing I should do is immobilize myself. He prescribed exercises and deep breathing to get the circulation going and oxygen flowing and to make me relax. They are meditation-type exercises that I do when I feel muscle tension coming on. Sometimes I lie flat on my back on the office floor and breathe deeply.

"I've begun exercising again, walking 4 or 5 miles, 2 to 3 times a week, and cycling on a stationary bike at least 12 miles a week. I also do bent-knee sit-ups, holding the position for 5 seconds.

"All of this has helped. I'm not saying the pain won't come back, because I am a very stressed person. But I have it under control. I know what is causing it, so now I have something to fight. According to Dr. Sarno, that is the key."

TEST YOUR BACK

Toronto back doctor David Imrie, M.D., author of *Goodbye Backache,* has devised this simple, 4-exercise test to tell you if muscle weakness and joint stiffness is causing your back pain now, or if it might in the future. Remember, this is a test to tell you what muscles you need to strengthen, not an exercise program. And should you feel any pain or strain, stop immediately.

The Sit-Up

This exercise determines the flexibility of your back and the strength of your stomach muscles. Lie on your back and bend your knees at a 45-degree angle. Place your hands behind your neck. Slowly and smoothly, sit up, keeping your feet flat on the floor. Don't jerk up and don't have someone hold your feet. If you can't sit up, place your arms across your chest and try again. If you still fail, try with your arms out straight.

Double Straight-Leg Raise

This determines stomach muscle strength. Lie face-up with your hands under the hollow of your back. Eliminate the hollow by tightening your stomach muscles and forcing your back flat against your hands and the floor. Raise both feet together 10 inches and hold for a 10 count, keeping your back flat on the floor. If you feel pain or your back curves, do not continue.

	The Sit-Up	Double Straight-Leg Raise
LEVEL 1	Able to sit up with knees bent and hands behind the neck.	Able to keep the back flat while raising the legs for 10 seconds.
EXCELLENT	Adequate spinal flexibility and abdominal strength.	Can demonstrate balanced pelvic position and hold it under extreme stress.
LEVEL 2	Able to sit up with knees bent and arms folded across chest.	Able to raise the legs for several seconds, but back curves partway through the test.
AVERAGE	Need to improve abdominal muscle strength.	Can achieve balanced pelvic position, but need more abdominal muscle strength for good posture under stress.
LEVEL 3	Able to sit up with knees bent and arms held out straight.	Able to lift the legs, but back curves as soon as legs are raised.
FAIR	Need to improve spinal flexibility and abdominal strength.	Need training in balanced pelvic position and increased abdominal strength.
LEVEL 4	Unable to sit up with knees bent.	Unable to lift both legs.
POOR	Need a great deal of improvement in both strength and flexibility.	Need extensive training in balanced pelvic position and increased abdominal strength.

Lateral Trunk Lift

This exercise tests the strength of trunk and leg muscles. Lie on your right side, legs straight. Fold your arms across your chest. Have someone firmly hold your feet down by the ankles. Slowly raise your upper body off the floor as far as possible and hold for a 10 count. Repeat on the left side. If there is pain or discomfort, stop the test. Do not jerk the body up or push up from the elbow. This invalidates the test. Your body must be perfectly straight while lying on your side.

Hip Flexors

These test the stretching power of hip flexing muscles. Lie face-up with your legs straight. Bend your right knee, grasp it, and bring it tight against your chest. Hold it, and determine the position of your left leg. Is it flat or raised? Repeat with the left leg. Remember, your head must remain on the floor and your knee must be held snugly to your chest. The critical upward movement of the extended leg occurs during the last part of the test.

Summing It Up

Using the chart below, circle the grade achieved in each test, then total your score.

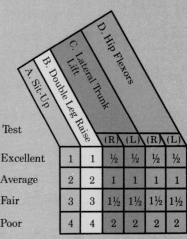

Test	A. Sit-Up	B. Double Leg Raise	C. Lateral Trunk Lift (R)	(L)	D. Hip Flexors (R)	(L)
Excellent	1	1	½	½	½	½
Average	2	2	1	1	1	1
Fair	3	3	1½	1½	1½	1½
Poor	4	4	2	2	2	2

NOTE: If you are over 45, subtract 2 to reach your total score.

Back Fitness Rating
4 to 5 = Excellent; 6 to 9 = Average; 10 to 13 = Fair; 14 to 16 = Poor.

If your score is less than excellent, you've got some work to do to prevent back problems. Talk to your doctor about exercises to strengthen your weak spots.

Lateral Trunk Lift	Hip Flexors
Able to raise the upper body 12 inches off the floor and hold for 10 count.	Able to bring knee completely to chest while keeping opposite leg flat on the floor.
Adequate lateral trunk muscles.	Hip flexors are all right.
Able to raise the upper body with difficulty and unable to hold for 10 count.	Able to bring knee to chest but other leg lifts slightly off the floor.
Need improvement in lateral trunk muscles.	Need to slightly stretch hip flexors.
Able to raise the upper body a few inches only and unable to hold.	Leg lifts completely off the floor when knee is pulled to chest.
Need improvement in lateral trunk muscles.	Need much improvement in hip flexors' stretching ability.
Unable to raise the body off the floor.	Leg flies up into the air when knee is held against chest.
Need much improvement in lateral trunk muscles.	Inadequate stretch in hip flexors—they need a great deal of stretching.

Proper Sit-Ups for Pain-Free Backs

Strong stomach muscles are vital to defeating back pain because they give the spine support and help the back muscles handle physical strain. Physical therapist Marilyn L. Miller, of Neskowin, Oregon, has developed these stomach-strengthening techniques that are especially good for back pain sufferers.

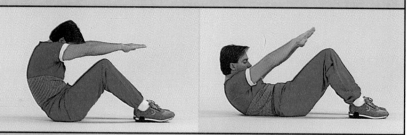

The Curl-Back

Sit on the floor with your knees bent, back rounded, and arms out front. Bend your head forward and contemplate your navel. Slowly uncurl your back, keeping your eyes on your navel and your heels on the floor. Breathe out to contract your abdominals as your back touches the floor slowly, one vertebra at a time. Stretch your arms behind you as you hit the floor and unbend your head. Take a deep breath. Aim for a smooth, 5-second motion.

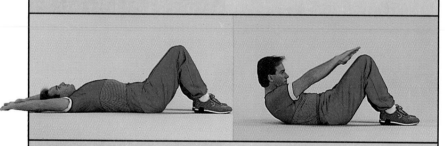

The Curl-Up

This is the reverse of the Curl-Back. Lie flat, with your knees bent and your arms on the floor above your head. Suck in your abdominals, exhale and let your arms lead you smoothly forward until you are curled, with your arms forward and your eyes on your navel.

When you can curl up without having your feet fly, you're ready to combine both curls into one motion. Breathe out as you curl back, take a breath, then breathe out again as you curl up. When it becomes easy, place your hands over your chest to give you more of a challenge and more of a reward.

strong stomach muscles.

Exercises aimed at the stomach, such as bent-knee sit-ups (see "Proper Sit-Ups for Pain-Free Backs" will help keep you painlessly erect.

MYTHICAL CAUSES OF BACK PAIN

If your doctor starts talking about one leg being shorter than the other, chances are he's groping. This often-diagnosed cause of back pain has little backing among today's medical community.

"Our doctors don't recommend lifts (shoe inserts that even leg lengths) unless there's a severe leg difference due to polio," says C. James Greenwood, Jr., M.D., former chief of neurosurgery and neurology at Baylor College of Medicine, Houston.

That's because several doctors have shown that legs that differ in length by as much as ½ inch are normal and probably do not cause back pain. According to the American Medical Association, "Most physicians believe that a difference of half an inch or less is probably insignificant." Despite this, some practitioners may continue to prescribe a trip to the shoemaker for ¼- to ½-inch lifts. If you have one and it hasn't helped, consider retiring it. If you're told to get one, get a second opinion instead.

SEX AND THE BAD BACK

Businessmen say the three most important aspects of retail business are location, location and location. To turn this truism around a bit, the three most important aspects of sex and backache are position, position and position.

There's no way around it: Sex involves the back, and the onset of back pain can doom the sex life of a couple unless they are willing to try new, pain-free positions.

The widely used missionary position may strain the man's muscles, especially if he arches his back. If the man has the bad back, one solution is to have the woman on top. Other popular alternatives are lying side by side facing each other, or stomach to back in the "spoon" position.

David Fardon, M.D., an orthopedic surgeon and physician at the Knoxville Back Care Center and founder of the Knoxville Orthopedic Clinic, gives this advice to women with back pain who want to use the missionary position: "Place a pillow under your hips and lower back. Bend the knees. This is a satisfactory positon for sexual intercourse and an ideal position for a sore back.

"You don't have to swear off sex because of back pain," assures Dr. Fardon. "Sexual activity and the back are related only in position and movement. There is nothing about erection and ejaculation or penetration of the female pelvis that should cause trouble with the back."

EXERCISING THE DEMON

You don't have to swear off exercise, either. Exercise aimed at firming up the back and stomach muscles can ease current back pain or prevent future pain for many people. But before you start, a word of caution: Dr. Hendler believes that because back pain can have a variety of causes, some bone, disk or structural problems can be intensified by exercise. "Patients should have an individual exercise program devised by their doctor," he says. Once you've been given your doctor's okay, it's best to stay within the limits of your pain by easing into a program that decreases the pain over a period of time.

Dr. Fardon and his clinic director, physical therapist Cathy Shope, have their patients exercise as soon as the problem has been diagnosed.

"Two good ones are the pelvic tilt and the standing pelvic tilt because they help your posture as well as your back muscles," Ms. Shope says.

Dr. Fardon and Ms. Shope give these instructions for exercises to build up your back and relieve pain.

The Pelvic Tilt. "Lie down on your back. Bend your knees and put your feet flat. Relax your arms at your sides. Tighten your buttock muscles together as though trying to hold a coin between them. Now tighten your abdominal muscles so that your back lies flat on the floor, eliminating the normal pocket of space formed by the

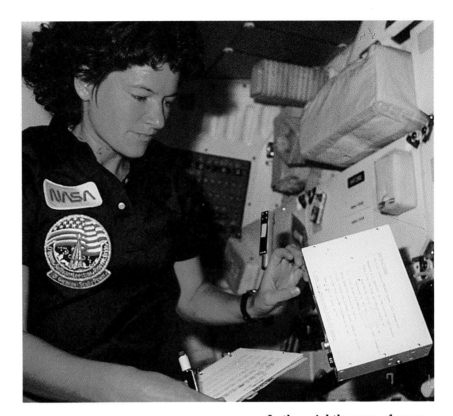

arch of your back. Your stomach should be sucked in and your pelvic bone tilting upward. Progress over time to the point of actually lifting your buttocks up an inch or two from the floor without allowing your back to rise."

The Standing Pelvic Tilt. "Stand with your back to a wall with your hips, heels and shoulders touching the wall. Feel the space formed between the arch of your lower back and the wall. Suck in your stomach, tighten your buttock muscles, tilt your pelvis and reduce the space by pushing your back flat against the wall. Feel yourself 'getting tall' as your back straightens.

"You should hold these exercises for about 5 seconds and do them five to ten times each," Dr. Fardon says.

Dr. Lehrman also emphasizes exercise and includes the quadricep stretch in his program to relieve back pain.

The Quadricep Stretch. "Stand about 3 feet from a wall and extend your left arm to the wall to support your body. Reach down with your right hand and grab your right ankle or foot. Gently pull your heel toward your

In the weightlessness of space, astronauts often "grow" as much as 2 inches. This is because the jellylike spinal nucleus is no longer squashed by body weight, enabling it to expand. (The first spacesuits didn't allow for this growth and drew complaints from irritated astronauts.) The same expansion happens when you sleep, though it's not nearly as dramatic.

buttocks. Do a pelvic tilt to prevent your back from sagging. Hold for 30 seconds. Repeat three to five times with each leg," says Dr. Lehrman.

THE SPORTING BACK

There's another type of exercise that's okay for your back: sports. "Even the most vigorous sports activities won't harm your back," says Hamilton Hall, M.D., of Toronto General Hospital. "They may simply make it hurt for a few days . . . [but] hurt is not the same as harm, and the trade-off may be worth it."

"That's good advice," agrees Hubert L. Rosomoff, M.D., professor and chairman of the department of neurosurgery and medical director of the Comprehensive Pain Center at the University of Miami Medical School. "Sports can't harm the back. We never advise anyone to give up the sports they like," he says. "We get them back to playing or back to work, even if it's heavy labor. However, there are certain things we don't like. Jogging is bad for people who have injured the lower parts of their bodies. Swimming is excellent, as is rowing. A brisk walk with weights in the hands, like Heavyhands, is also good for the back.

"If you become sore from an exercise or activity that you haven't done in a while, don't worry. Routine soreness is nothing to fear. Depending on your original condition, the soreness should be gone in 12 to 72 hours. If it lasts longer than that, you may need some help, so a visit to your doctor is advised," Dr. Rosomoff says.

Dr. Hall adds that weight-bearing sports like weight lifting and bowling may cause excessive straining, so be careful. Golf and racquet sports involve a lot of rotation that can heighten existing pain, so you might want to adjust your swings. Although cycling hunches you over, Dr. Hall says it could be a good sport for chronic back pain sufferers. Bike riding induces the pelvic tilt, which takes the stress off the back and allows the legs and other lower body muscles to be exercised. (People with disk diseases should consult their doctors before riding a bike.)

Dr. Tessman advises back pain sufferers to avoid exercising for the first 15 minutes after a night's sleep. "I realize many people immediately launch into an exercise program to help wake up, but this can be harmful," he says. "The fluids have collected in the disks of the spine after sleeping, and this makes you more vulnerable to strains and other injuries."

WHITE PARCELS OF PAIN RELIEF?

But what if self-help techniques *don't* work? Is a little white pill the answer? One expert doesn't think so.

"Drugs rarely help at all," Dr. Rosomoff states flatly. "They distort perception and make people think

The Right Bed for Your Back

Goldilocks was no dummy. She looked until she found the bed that was "just right." You should follow suit, because beds that are too soft place excessive strain on the muscles in the back. In fact, for some people, a too-soft bed may be the primary cause of back pain. The easiest way to stiffen your bed is to put a sheet of ¾-inch plywood under the entire mattress or put the mattress directly on the floor. When buying a bed, think firm. High-quality, firm mattresses are usually as good as expensive, "orthopedic" beds. Water and air mattresses also help some people.

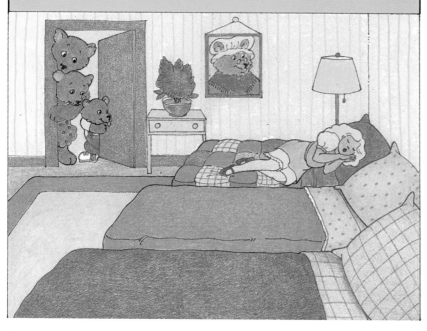

Shari Lewis
Beverly Hills, Calif.
Neck Pain

Lamb Chop was heartbroken. Hush Puppy was inconsolable. Even Charley Horse felt off his feed. Their best friend, diminutive dynamo Shari Lewis, was tormented by severe neck pain, a pain so relentless it reached into her magical fantasy world. It also reached into the 52-year-old star's other world, the one where she's an acclaimed stage actress, singer and dancer, a best-selling author and traveling symphony conductor. With a schedule like that, there was no room for neck pain. In the 5-time Emmy Award winner's own words, this is how she got it and how she beat it.

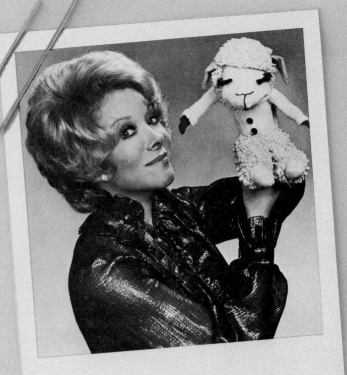

"As a dancer, you often expose yourself to the cold when you're soaking with sweat after vigorous routines. A few years ago I was performing in a stage play in San Francisco. The dressing room was a cold, damp, basement dungeon. I came in dripping wet after a scene, got hit with the cold, and developed neuralgia [nerve pain]. I spent 6 weeks in sheer agony, but I couldn't stop. I had to break in a new Vegas routine at a club in Hot Springs, Arkansas. I was in such misery that my musical director contacted the head of a nearby veterans' hospital. The doctor put me on a program that has been a lifesaver:

"Whenever I feel the pain coming on, the first thing I do is take an ice-cold bottle of Coke and place it at the back of my neck, using it for a pillow. I keep it there until it becomes uncomfortable—no specific amount of time.

"Then I do the following exercise routine every day. First, I stand with my shoulders relaxed and turn my head to the right as far as I can, then left. I do this (and all the following exercises) 20 times each way.

"Then I move my head sideways, bringing my ear down to my shoulder, stretching the opposite side of my neck.

"The next exercise is 'The Turtle.' I keep my chin level with the floor, lift my shoulders up and pull my head in like a turtle. I alternate this by stretching the top of the back of my head up toward the ceiling, keeping my shoulders down.

"Next, I relax my arms and rotate my shoulders in circles, 20 times back and 20 times forward.

"Finally, I stand facing into a corner. I place my hands shoulder high on the wall on each side and do pushups, pushing my nose to the wall and back out.

"The first time I did all this, the pain disappeared in 24 hours!"

And that means all is well in Lamb Chop's world again.

When to See a Doctor for Neck Pain

As many as 9 in 10 cases of chronic neck pain may be due to muscle contractions or tension. That's good news because it means there is no structural or permanent damage to be alarmed about. However, there are times when neck pain *can* signal serious trouble. These are the warnings that should send you immediately to a doctor: pain traveling down an arm; a numb or tingly arm; pain in your neck along with fever and headache; a neck so stiff that the chin can't be touched to the chest.

they have pain that is far greater than they have. Drugs distort judgment, too, and they knock you out. Muscle relaxants have no effect whatsoever in the usual dosage. They are only effective at the point of toxicity. None of the pain-relieving drugs actually cure pain. If you must use something, simple aspirin remains the best medication to take."

NO MORE NECK PAIN

Doctors label it a separate part, but the neck is simply one of the top rungs on the body's ladder. And like back pain, almost all neck pain is caused by simple stress and tension—two opponents you can beat without expensive medical care, according to Dr. John Sarno of New York University Medical Center. Once your doctor has eliminated the possibility of major physical problems, you can fight your neck pain with relaxation techniques and exercise.

That's why the best doctor for your neck may well be the fictional Dr. Marcus Welby. In a popular commercial playing off his healer image, actor Robert Young implores frantic people to relax. In the real world, Dr. Fardon recommends relaxation techniques for neck pain.

"Meditation is an excellent way to relax," he advises. "It's also easy. Just sit in a comfortable position and concentrate on your breathing. And don't be uptight about trying to keep other thoughts out of your head. Just let them go by as you focus on your breathing.

"A second method is what is called guided imagery," he says. "Visualize your neck pain in terms of an image or object. Think of it as, say, a red lightning bolt. Then slowly allow the colors to fade from red to orange to yellow to a cool, soft blue. The point is to change it from a sharp to a soft image. Do this every time you feel the pain until you have fully identified your image as the pain. Then you can fade it out every time."

Stanley Grosshandler, M.D., medical director of the Raleigh Pain Clinic and associate professor of anesthesia at the University of North Carolina, says sufferers may also need to fade out real stress from their lives.

"Work out your problems about why you hate your boss or why you are mad at your wife," he says. "Settle that lawsuit about your auto accident and get it off your mind. Get this extra stress out of your neck! If you can't do it yourself, a pain clinic psychologist who is experienced in the treatment of pain can help."

"Get rid of your fear," adds Dr. Rosomoff. "Fear is a huge enemy, especially fear about the pain itself. Doctors are guilty of scaring the life out of their patients by talking about wheelchairs and paralysis. In most cases this is unfounded. Be confident that the pain can be eliminated through exercise and proper care."

TWISTING AND TURNING

Internationally famous entertainer Shari Lewis details the exercises that work for her neck on page 21. Thorough as her routine is, there are other exercises doctors recommend.

"Stretching the jaw muscles can ease pain and tension in the neck," Dr. Fardon says. "You can do this simply by opening your mouth as wide as you can a few times and holding it open for a few seconds.

"Watch out for clenched teeth. This is a sign of stress and possible neck problems. The only times your teeth should ever clench is when you swallow. The rest of the time, make sure your teeth are apart. Let the jaw slack a bit. If it is tight, do the stretching exercise," he recommends.

"Another good stretching exercise is to pull your shoulder blades back together by pulling the shoulders back. Do this a few times to loosen up. You can also tighten and loosen your shoulder and neck muscles. This allows you to become mentally conscious of them, and helps teach you to relax.

"For extratight muscles, you can apply some heat in the form of a hot cloth or towel prior to exercise. Use ice on injured or strained muscles to aid in healing," Dr. Fardon adds.

Exercise scientist Michael Wolf, Ph.D., of New York, adds a rotation exercise to Ms. Lewis's routine.

"Swing your head over to one shoulder, come back down around the front and over to the other shoulder and back to center. This should all be done slowly, gradually, within pain-free limits. If you hear some cracks and pops, don't worry. That's the natural process of gas coming out of the solution in the joints. If there is specific pain directly associated with the cracks, then you should see a doctor," he says.

If you're knotted up from hunching over office or school work, Harold Gelb, D.M.D., of the University of Medicine and Dentistry of New Jersey, suggests you "shrug your shoulders as high as you can and then let them go. Do a few head rolls. Sit back in your chair and take a deep breath. Exhale and let your whole body go limp. . . . During a stressful period, try to break away from what you're doing and take a few deep breaths."

RUB OUT PAIN

"A simple light massage from a partner or friend can relieve tightness or tension and bring blood to the region," Dr. Wolf advises. "Don't worry about precise techniques. Rubbing the muscles and kneading them slightly will work. Just do it smoothly, rhythmically and gently."

Despite some problems you may encounter getting a correct diagnosis from a doctor, the overall picture regarding neck pain is optimistic. Self-care is the key.

"The human body is a marvelous machine with safety and corrective mechanisms built into it. With a little instruction, you should be able to maintain a pain-free neck and back all your life," says Los Angeles physical therapist Hyman Jampol.

Notice he said instruction, not prescription. Drugs seem to be falling out of favor in the war against neck pain. The once-popular muscle relaxants are taking it on the chin the most as numerous doctors, including Dr. Rosomoff and Dr. Grosshandler, question their value. Powerful painkillers are also being criticized because they have a potential for abuse and adverse side effects and offer only temporary relief from pain.

If you must take medication, aspirin remains the best for both neck and back problems.

How to Relieve Your Stiff Neck

The report was due yesterday. Your secretary quit and the IRS won't. You've developed a whopper of a stiff neck. Now relieve it.

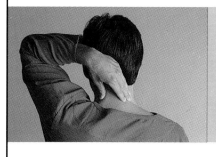

1. Grab the back of your neck with one hand by placing your fingers on one side and your thumb on the other. Draw the fingers and thumb toward each other until they are an inch apart on either side of the spine. The muscle you feel is the trapezius muscle.

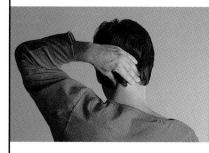

2. Work the fingers and thumb gently up along the muscle into the hairline as if you were fluting the edge of a piecrust.

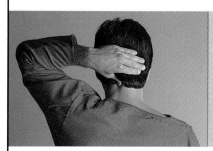

3. If you find a sensitive spot, press it as hard as the pain allows for 10 seconds. Then release the pressure slowly.

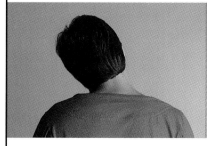

4. Stretch the trapezius muscle by bending your head forward, then to the right, lowering your ear toward your shoulder. Then bend it to the left. Repeat steps 1 to 4, paying attention to the sensitive spots.

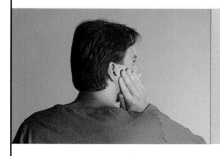

5. Put your right hand on your cheek and turn your head to the right, giving gentle resistance with the hand. Repeat, moving to the left.

Repeat 1 to 5 times every 2 hours until you feel relaxed.

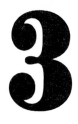

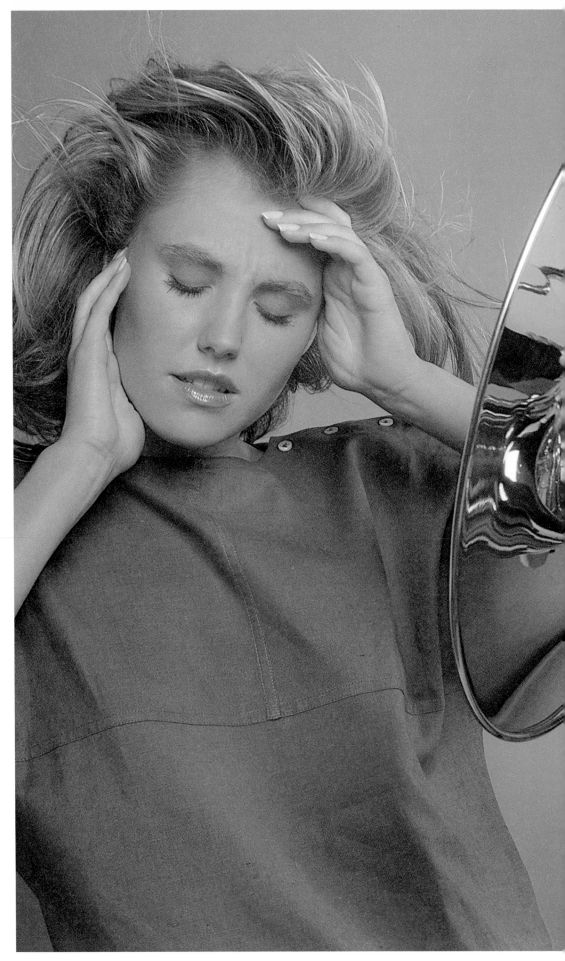

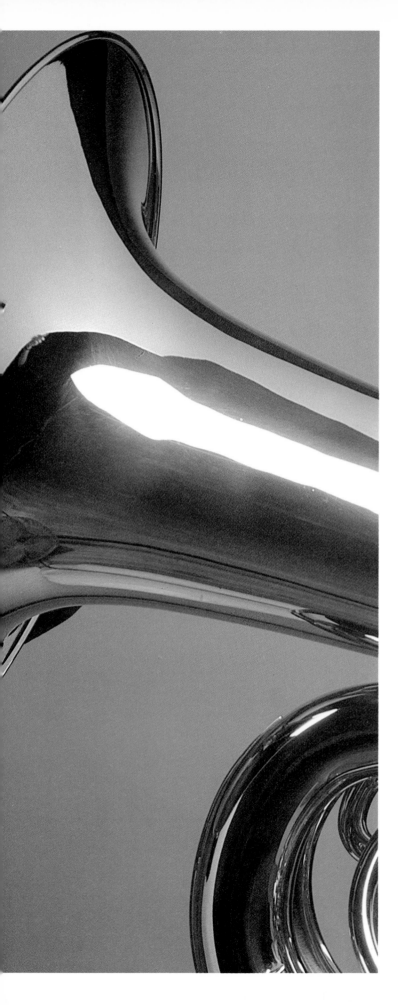

Freedom from Headache Pain

Don't let headaches sneak up and knock you out. Fight back with these moves—and win.

She actually considered looking in the mirror to see if it was visible. The steel band had tightened around her forehead. Her temples pounded against the metal. "Surely you ought to be able to see something that hurts so much," she thought. But if Laura had looked into the mirror, all she would have seen was the *effect* of the pain—her face drained of color, eyes half closed, brow furrowed—not the *cause*, a full-blown tension headache.

People who suffer from serious headache pain often describe it in torturous detail, calling up images of hot pokers plunged into eye sockets, grenades exploding behind the forehead, sinuses stuffed with ice-cold, quick-setting cement. Medieval dungeon masters could have taken lessons from those who suffer head pain.

Every day millions of people are tormented with pain that can last hours or days, occur every week or twice a year, hurt like a minor buzzing or a knife plunged into the brain. The suffering can be of such savage intensity that victims may feel the easiest way to get relief would be to tear off their own heads.

One might suspect that pain this vicious would be rare. Not so.

- Ninety percent of us will suffer headaches in some degree at least once. For some, this pain is a way of life that has to be coped with, or just endured, on a daily basis.

- About 30 million Americans suffer from headaches and an additional 15 million live with the constant threat of migraine attacks—that's one-fifth of the population.

Why Your Head Aches

If you think a headache is caused by brain pain, think again. That headache's not in your brain or skull.

The constant, whole-head pain of tension headaches is from tense, constricted muscles in the face, jaw, neck and scalp. The less common but often more excruciating vascular headaches (migraine, cluster) cause a throbbing pain when blood vessels swell.

- The labor lost due to severe, disabling headaches equals 124 million workdays a year, costing $6.2 billion.
- Headache sufferers spend $8.4 billion a year in search of relief; headache and migraine remedies account for $1.2 billion of that amount.

But much of this expense and suffering is unnecessary. There are lots of ways to have relief from headaches—many as simple as cutting back on certain foods or learning effective ways to relax. *You* can learn to be headache free.

ONE HEAD—MANY PAINS!

The term *headache* covers a variety of ills affecting the head, face, neck and even shoulders. But our most common perception of a headache is a feeling of pain actually inside the head, even deep within the brain.

A surprising fact to most people is that the brain itself is impervious to pain. The double-fist-sized organ which controls our whole being is a gelatinous mass of gray matter that feels nothing. You could beat, smash, pound, pummel and puncture the brain, but you'd still experience no pain.

What, then, accounts for the pain we feel? Ninety percent of all persistent headaches are caused by tension in the muscles of the head and neck, according to one of the country's leading headache and migraine specialists, Seymour Diamond, M.D., of the Diamond Headache Clinic in Chicago. These clenched muscles are frequently the result of tension, stress or depression.

Migraines and cluster headaches, on the other hand, are caused by expansion of the blood vessels in the head. Enlarged, says Dr. Diamond, they apply pressure on sensitive nerves, causing pain. These blood vessels can dilate in reaction to certain foods, alcohol, excessive smoking and (in women) hormonal changes.

RELAX PAIN AWAY

Tension headaches are easy to identify because of their dull, bandlike, persistent pain that often encompasses the whole head. They may last for several hours and can occur on a daily basis or several times a month. While they're painful, they needn't dominate your life. You can get rid of them with simple, effective self-help methods. Over-the-counter painkillers like aspirin offer relief to those who have only occasional tension headaches. To counter more frequent headaches, try teaching yourself to relax. This can be as easy as sitting or lying back, closing your eyes and just resting for an hour while your thoughts wander.

And anything you can do at home to relax your head, neck and facial muscles will probably help your headache. Apply heat to tensed neck muscles. Soak in a hot tub or take a steaming bath, with your neck and the back of your head submerged. Or talk a friend into giving you a soothing massage, as discussed in chapter 8.

You also can learn tension- and stress-relaxation techniques such as biofeedback, which can both prevent and relieve headaches—particularly for people who suffer daily tension headaches. Your local hospital is likely to be a good source for group classes or relaxation specialists in your area.

TENSE SLEEP

Sleep should be relaxing, but it's often a cause of headache. You might be getting too little sleep, or you could even be catching too many Z's. Take a look at your regular sleep patterns and see if they are being disrupted in any way. That occasional extra-early morning wake-up might turn out to be the root cause of your occasional headache. Or, if you find yourself with a headache on weekends when you sleep late, try cutting back on those long lay-ins.

Another good method of relieving pain is described in "Press Head Pain Away," on page 29. A similar technique, acupressure, also often helps. If these self-cure remedies don't relieve your tension headaches, you might require professional help. Your doctor can advise you about which drugs are best for your tension headache.

Donald Cupertino
Bronxville, N.Y.
Tension Headache

A scene from nearly 4 years ago: Perspiration dampened Donald Cupertino's dark brown hair as his head began to pound. Normally poised and good looking, the 27-year-old funeral director from Bronxville, New York, grew pale and queasy in the Atlantic City sunshine. "Oh, God," he sighed, as the familiar pain threatened his long-awaited vacation. "Another day is ruined."

Three years previously, Donald was in perfect health. He got occasional headaches, but a couple of aspirins always stopped the pain. However, around the time his first child was born, the headaches became intensely painful and more frequent. He'd often wake up to a dull hammering behind his eyes. As the day wore on, the pain would increase to a steady, rhythmic throbbing, with knifelike stabs punctuating the hammer blows. Eventually, the headaches became a daily nightmare, and neither aspirin nor sleep could stop the pain. Donald grew afraid that he had a brain tumor.

His doctor prescribed Fiorinal, a muscle relaxant that worked only when Donald took it round-the-clock. A dentist diagnosed TMJ disorder, a defect in his jaw alignment, and recommended a chiropractor. Ten spinal adjustments later, he still had the headaches.

In desperation, he saw a neurologist, who ruled out a tumor but still found no cause for the headaches. Finally, exasperated by the headache in Atlantic City, Donald followed a friend's suggestion and called the headache unit at Montefiore Hospital in the Bronx for help.

At Montefiore, the problem was diagnosed as chronic muscle tension headaches. Biofeedback, he was told, would teach him how to actually relax his

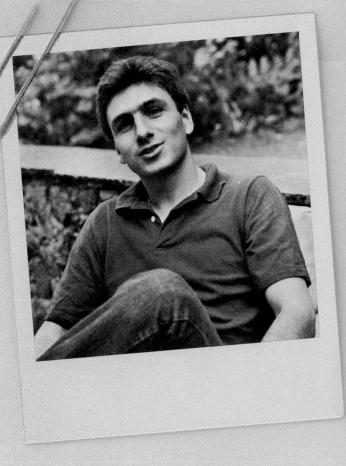

overworked muscles and alleviate the pain. Once a week, a skeptical Donald was wired to a temperature gauge and an electromyogram machine. Electrodes on his forehead and hand monitored his muscle tension, which he tried to lower with deep breathing and relaxation techniques. All the while he monitored his progress on the biofeedback equipment. He practiced the regimen at home and began to implement the exercises in his daily life. His muscles began to register less tension.

After only 8 weeks, the headaches were nearly gone. The few he still gets are minor compared to the unbearable throbbing he felt in Atlantic City. He can often cut them short with the relaxation techniques he mastered at Montefiore. "The biofeedback changed my life," Donald says gratefully. "It's a good feeling not to have the pain anymore."

Fever Headaches

Fever headaches occur when unwanted bacteria release toxins into the bloodstream that cause the body's temperature to rise. This makes blood vessels swell, giving you a throbbing headache.

When headaches caused by fever persist even when you take aspirin or other simple analgesics, put an ice pack on the site of the pain—a throbbing temple, for example—for relief.

Another, rarer kind of stress headache is due to eyestrain. Such headaches usually start at the front of the head and can spread across a wide band covering both sides of the skull.

Eyestrain headaches can be triggered by muscle imbalance, uncorrected vision or astigmatism. If you have no luck treating your headache and it fits the description above, have your doctor recommend an eye specialist. Something as simple as reading glasses might be the instant answer.

But tension and strain aren't the only reasons people get headaches. Other common causes include allergies, head congestion, exercise and food sensitivity.

Allergy Headache. These headaches are a direct result of seasonal allergens such as pollens and molds.

Along with headache, the symptoms include nasal congestion and watery eyes. Treatments include antihistamines and allergy shots.

Sinus Headache. Sometimes headache-causing congestion is present when allergies aren't. Such is the case with sinus headaches—a gnawing pain in the nasal area or forehead that can become more severe as the day goes on. The pain is due to blocked sinus ducts that prevent normal drainage, and may be accompanied by acute infection and fever. Swelling and tenderness around the forehead, nose and cheeks are common.

Sinus headaches are rare, but you can treat them by inhaling moist heat from a warm, wet towel or the steam from a basin of hot water. OTC analgesics also help. And ask your doctor for drugs that treat inflammation and infection and drain clogged sinuses.

Workout Headache. Heavy exercise can aggravate headache pain. The pain comes when the smaller blood vessels don't expand fast enough to handle stepped-up blood supply from the exercise.

Don't take this type of headache lightly, however. Although 90 percent of these headaches are not serious (most often they are the result of headaches already in progress), 10 percent are caused by exercise and

may be related to serious problems, including aneurysms, tumors or blood vessel malformation. If you think the problem might be serious, don't mess around with this one—seek professional medical help immediately. Otherwise, just take things a little easier.

Hunger Headache. Exactly as its name suggests, the hunger headache is the body's natural response to lack of food. The pain strikes just before regular mealtimes and may be caused by muscle tension, low blood sugar or swelling of blood vessels due to excessive dieting or skipping meals. Sometimes it's easy to forget to eat when you are swamped with work or other obligations. The best cure is to eat a meal or a snack.

Food-Sensitivity Headache. Just the opposite of the hunger headache, it's caused by foods that you may be sensitive to.

More specialists now realize that a significant number of headaches can be traced directly to diet. Samuel Seltzer, D.D.S., and Robert Pollack, Ph.D., of Temple University in Philadelphia, say that 5 percent of their head and neck pain patients can trace their problem back to foods they eat.

Dr. Pollack, a biochemist and nutritionist, reveals, "We have managed to identify 25 separate pain syndromes caused directly by substances we eat or drink." Many of these pains are in the head.

The logic behind the food-sensitivity headache makes perfect sense. Certain foods, once absorbed into the bloodstream, act to either constrict or dilate blood vessels in the head, resulting in headaches. But not everybody is affected by *each food* in the same way. What's good for the goose may not be good for the gander.

The most effective way to test for a food sensitivity is to make a note of when your headaches occur and recall what foods you ate prior to the headache. Since most of these diet offenders act swiftly, often producing symptoms within 45 minutes of being consumed, it's not too difficult to tell what meal triggered the problem. Next time you have the same meal, eliminate one of the possible edible adversaries, testing foods one by one until you find the culprit. For example: If you get a headache after eating a grilled cheese sandwich, french fries and a chocolate shake, try eliminating the french fries next time. If you still get a headache, that means the french fries were not to blame and next time you should skip the grilled cheese. If you still get the headache, try eliminating the shake next. Keep eliminating until you find the culprit food and then avoid it.

Here is a list of the most common problem foods, drinks and additives: smoked fish, pickled herring, shellfish, bologna, salami, pepperoni, bacon, frankfurters, corned beef, canned ham, chopped liver, cheese (especially aged or smoked cheddars), canned figs, lima or string beans, yeast, chocolate, nutmeg, licorice (natural, not artificial), hard liquor, beer, red wine (especially Chianti), champagne, coffee (not decaffeinated), tea and some herbal teas.

Caffeine Headache. Caffeine is found in a lot of foods and is responsible for a lot of headaches. Caffeine in moderation may relieve headaches in some people by narrowing already widened vessels (for this reason, it is in many OTC painkillers), but it also has a rebound effect when overused.

This type of rebound headache hits people who drink a lot of coffee, tea or cola during the week— typically five to ten cups a day—but hardly ever touch the stuff on the weekend. Suddenly stopping the supply of caffeine on Saturday and Sunday can have adverse results as the body suffers from withdrawal symptoms. Blood vessels, normally used to a slight narrowing from caffeine, swell and begin to pound, leaving you in pain.

The most obvious cure for this problem is to gradually cut caffeine intake during the week, so you don't have a jolt on the weekend. Or have a cup on Saturday morning to keep your system adjusted.

CLUSTER HEADACHES

Cluster headaches are in a class by themselves. They can rival and even

Press Head Pain Away

To relieve your headache with pressure, first relax, close your eyes and conjure up a pleasing mental image.

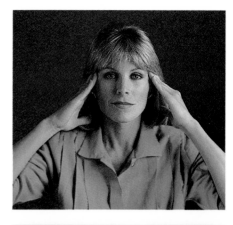

Place the three middle fingers of each hand on your temples, above and in front of your ears.

Gently apply pressure with one finger at a time, moving each around to probe for sensitive points. When you find one, increase the pressure slightly for 10 seconds and then slowly release it.

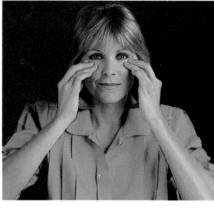

Next, do the same thing on the bony area of your eye sockets, both above and below your eyes.

Next, run your fingers through your hair and along your scalp in a rhythmic head massage.

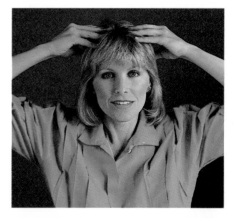

Rest and repeat, if needed. Then slide the tip of an ice cube around your forehead in short swipes, always going in the same direction.

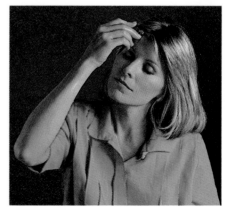

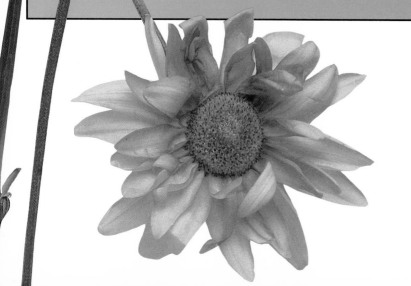

Dos and Don'ts of a Hangover Headache

To avoid pain the morning after:

Do

- Eat oil- or fat-rich foods before drinking. Peanut butter or cheeses are ideal. So is a glass of milk.
- Space out your intake of alcohol over a long period of time.
- Drink plenty of orange juice or any other vitamin-C-rich drink before bed.
- Take a simple painkiller like acetaminophen at bedtime.
- Settle your stomach in the morning with an antacid.

Don't

- Drink to excess.
- Drink carbonated drinks. They increase the rate at which alcohol is absorbed.
- Take aspirin, because it can further irritate your stomach lining.
- Try a "hair of the dog" cocktail the morning after. It masks the symptoms only briefly and makes the hangover worse.

exceed the woes of migraine for sheer unadulterated pain.

Clusters strike with sudden severity and little or no warning, and usually last from 30 minutes to 3 hours. Their name comes from the fact that they recur a number of times a day for as long as 12 months.

The mystery of these clusters is that they may suddenly vanish altogether and not reappear for months or years. They are totally unpredictable, and that's what makes them all the more devastating and difficult. This unpredictability can slowly but surely grind down even the strongest of wills.

Everything about cluster headaches is a puzzle, except the fact that clusters attack six times more men than women. The general profile of a cluster victim is a middle-aged man, a heavy smoker, with no history of blood-vessel-related headaches (even though cluster headache pain is definitely due to swollen blood vessels).

His headache will feel like this, according to Donald J. Dalessio, M.D., of Scripps Clinic and Research Foundation, La Jolla, California: "The one-sided pain is excruciating—burning and boring in character. It involves the region of the eye, the temple, the neck and often the face, and may extend into the shoulder on the involved side. It may also spread to the upper teeth and occasionally to the lower teeth.

"Cluster attacks, each usually lasting less than an hour and terminating as abruptly as they begin, often awaken the victim at night. The pain is so severe that he often jumps out of bed before he is fully awake," Dr. Dalessio explains.

Along with pain like that of a red-hot metal spike being pounded into the skull near the eye, there are other miserable symptoms, including tears flowing profusely, congestion that makes breathing difficult, a runny nose and heavy sweating.

The pain of cluster headaches is so vicious that 32 percent of cluster victims in one study admitted they wept during an attack; 37 percent yelled and screamed; 16 percent banged their heads against a wall, and 14 percent writhed on the floor. Some of the people in the study, conducted at the Faulkner Hospital in Boston, even admitted considering suicide as an escape from their agonies.

Finding relief from cluster headaches isn't easy, but it is possible. Because alcohol, heavy smoking, fatigue and stress can trigger cluster headaches, drink alcohol moderately, stop smoking and try getting enough sleep. If you still get the headaches, ask your doctor for ergotamine tartrate (a blood-vessel-constricting drug used in migraine treatments). If this does not help, several other medications are available that, when taken on a regular basis, can prevent the headaches from occurring.

Another effective treatment for cluster headaches is air—specifically, pure oxygen. "The results are spectacular," says Lee Kudrow, M.D., former editor of the medical journal *Headache.* After inhaling pure oxygen through a face mask for 15 minutes, his patients find relief from their cluster headaches. Your physician can help you with oxygen therapy and tell you how to use a home unit.

THE POWERFUL MIGRAINE

Migraines inspire fear and dread, just like cluster headaches. And like clusters, migraines are terrifying as much for their unpredictability as for their pain.

And the side effects that sometimes accompany migraine can be as shatteringly disturbing as the pain: wild visual displays; loss of coordination; vertigo; nausea; vomiting; and more. And the migraine can occur on different sides of your head. The name comes from the Latin for "half-skull," because the pain is usually in only one side of the head. But it also may strike one side in one attack and switch sides for the next one. It also might decide to hit both sides at once. And the migraine may be "classic" (with warning signs) or "common" (with no warning).

Migraine also has a sex bias: It attacks three times as many women as men. Migraine is to women what cluster headaches are to men.

A giant breakthrough in understanding migraine was made in the late 1960s when researchers pinpointed two major abnormalities that are common to migraine.

They found that blood flow through the brain decreases immediately prior to the headache phase of an attack and increases as the head pain begins to grow in ferocity; the cranial blood vessels constrict, increasing blood pressure, and then suddenly dilate, opening a floodgate of blood pounding through the head.

CLASSIC MIGRAINE

Of the two forms of migraine, classic and common, the classic is best known because it has its own peculiar warning system. First you enter a visually disoriented nightmare world of bizarre images, known in medical terms as the prodrome.

According to John Stirling Meyers, M.D., director of the cerebral blood-flow laboratories at the Veterans' Administration Medical Center in Houston and professor of neurology at Baylor College of Medicine, the prodrome lasts approximately 30 minutes and "usually consists of photopsias—scintillating flashing lights, lines or dots that may be yellow, gray, silver, grayish black or other colors.

The Rare Symptoms of Brain Tumors

The fear of a brain tumor often comes to mind when someones gets sudden or repeated headaches. This fear is usually unfounded.

In a study of 50 migraine sufferers at the National Hospital for Nervous Diseases in London, the biggest fear people had was of brain tumors. But they really had little reason to worry. Less than 1 percent of people who visit headache clinics are actually diagnosed as having brain tumors. And the symptoms are generally different from other head pains.

Chances are you don't have a brain tumor unless you have the following warning signs: headaches that become progressively worse over a short time; speech or personality changes; projectile vomiting; upset equilibrium, coordination or gait; seizures; drowsiness; increased pain when you cough, sneeze or change your physical position. Of course, if you're worried, it's always wise to see your doctor.

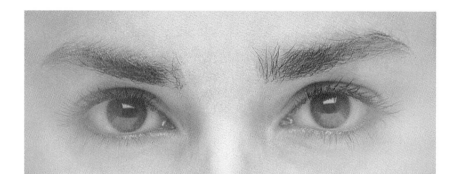

Migraine Warning Signals

The usual prodrome, or warning before a migraine, consists of one or more of the following symptoms: visual disturbances, including flashing lights, tunnel vision, blind spots, dimness, poor peripheral vision; distorted sense of smell, sound or taste; numbness; cold; feeling of pins and needles pricking the body; giddiness; muscle weakness; poor sense of balance; difficulty finding the right word when talking.

"These lines or dots move across or obscure the visual field so that the vision is impaired. Rarely, the prodrome may be characterized by numbness of one side of the body or around the mouth, or there may be weakness or clumsiness of one side of the body," he says.

Then the blood vessels dilate and the full migraine strikes like a sledgehammer. "And now comes the pain often one-sided, usually described as aching or throbbing, beating with the pulse, and sometimes eased when pressure is applied to the arteries," says Dr. Dalessio. He adds that often blood vessels become inflamed and sometimes swell. "By this time, the pain has incapacitated the sufferer, often with associated nausea and vomiting," he says. Many victims are unable to stand any stimulation, especially light (even dim light) and escape to a darkened room to endure the pain. A classic attack can last from 8 hours to several days. Often the victim falls asleep and then awakens to find the pain gone.

Classic migraine is not easy to live with. But common migraine is about as painful and may be even worse because it comes without the visual warning.

COMMON, BUT UNEXPECTED

Common migraines can literally hit you out of the blue.

"There is no definite prior indication of oncoming headache," explains Dr. Dalessio, "although some people say they can tell when the headache is coming by a vague change in mood, a 'feeling different,' just before" the onset of pain.

The pain of common migraine can be all-encompassing because it is usually on both sides of the head, rather than on just one side as with classic migraine.

And common migraine is more likely to be related to occupational, environmental or other stress, with some victims describing their condition as a food-related or a "premenstrual" headache, points out Dr. Dalessio. These last migraines are a common type.

WOMEN'S MIGRAINES

Migraines can be devastating—and all too familiar—for women, since 80 percent of migraine sufferers are women.

Because many of the attacks are associated with specific phases during the menstrual cycle, it is now widely held that these migraines may be linked to the body's delicate balance of female hormones.

The reason for this may be that the female hormone estrogen acts as a trigger for migraine attacks. Many women suffer more migraines while menstruating, and the incidence of migraine among women declines dramatically after menopause. Both phases involve shifting estrogen levels.

Scientists use hormone-based oral contraceptives to study this relationship between hormones and headaches.

Research with the Pill conducted by Robert E. Ryan, Sr., M.D., professor of otolaryngology at St. Louis University School of Medicine in Missouri, shows a definite connection between estrogen and migraine headaches. But the response is differ-

Sandra L.
Chicago, Ill.
Migraine

One of the best times of Sandra's life was when she was pregnant. And the ecstasy over the anticipated new arrival wasn't the sole reason!

Once pregnant, the young housewife suddenly found herself totally free of the agonizing migraine attacks that had plagued her for two long years.

The first migraine struck quite out of the blue when she was 17. It was followed immediately by 4 more in rapid succession that struck with all the devastation of a mental Mack truck.

"Sometimes I'd cry myself dry. All I'd want to do was lie there and die," recalls Sandra. "It wasn't just the incredible pain pounding away in my head; it also felt like my whole body was being put through a wringer that was trying to squeeze every bit of life out of me. This would go on for 10 to 12 hours."

Along with the blinding pain, Sandra's severe headaches were accompanied by all the symptoms of migraine, including severe nausea and vomiting.

After the first couple of attacks she learned to recognize the classic warning signals.

"About 20 minutes before the pain. I'd begin seeing zigzagging bright lines, sort of small at first, and then they'd expand across both eyes in an arc shape.

"Then any object I looked at that came inside the arc would bend and sway and start growing and shrinking. It was very scary. But even worse was knowing that there was no way I could avoid what was coming next," admits Sandra.

What did come next was a classic migraine attack, usually on the left side of her head, with the severest pounding centered around the temple.

During the 9 months Sandra was pregnant she did not experience a single attack. "It seemed like being pregnant was the ultimate migraine cure. I'd never felt better in my life," Sandra remembers.

But her migraine-free bliss was to be short-lived. What Sandra didn't know was that the medical experts had long recognized a distinct connection between the hormone changes of pregnancy and a decrease in the incidence of migraines.

So after her child was born and her levels of the hormone estrogen returned to normal, the migraines returned with a vengeance, sometimes 5 times a month. Sandra knew it was time to turn to professional help.

Following the advice of the National Migraine Foundation in Chicago, Sandra saw a migraine specialist. While routine laboratory tests and neurological scans showed no abnormalities, the doctor did learn that Sandra's mother had also suffered bouts of severe headaches as a teenager. He diagnosed her problem as classic migraine, which is often inherited.

Sandra's doctor prescribed an 80-milligram long-lasting capsule of propranolol daily. Propanolol is a drug used for cardiovascular disease that has also been found to be effective in up to 70 percent of migraine cases. She also was told to take a prescription combination tablet of ergotamine tartrate and caffeine immediately when she felt a migraine coming on. This vasoconstricting drug is highly effective in aborting migraine.

The therapy worked. Sandra sums up her new life like this: "It's wonderful. I finally feel I've gotten a handle on the problem. I know, like most migraine sufferers, that I'll never be completely cured, but I don't have that deathly fear of another attack.

"Now the migraines are negligible, and with the drugs I can avoid the pain and misery before it starts. That means I can enjoy a normal life."

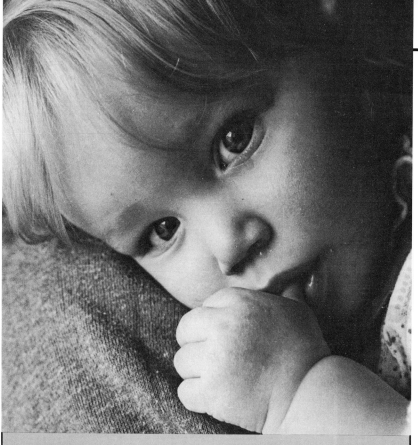

Relief for the Cruelest Headache

Almost 50 in every 1,000 children seen by pediatricians complain about throbbing, debilitating headaches, which are often accompanied by vomiting and occasionally by blurred vision, says Samuel J. Horwitz, M.D., associate professor of pediatrics and neurology at Case Western Reserve University, Cleveland.

Still, many doctors admit that childhood migraine is largely ignored in medical school training. But once the migraines are diagnosed, there is a safe, effective way to control them: biofeedback.

At the headache research and treatment center of the Menninger Foundation in Topeka, Kansas, 28 of 31 children, aged from 7 to 17 years, who suffered from migraine were able to successfully abort or control more than half of their attacks after taking a 2-month biofeedback and relaxation training course.

A similar biofeedback technique used in a small study by researchers at Louisiana State University showed the solution to be right at the kids' fingertips. With just 10 training sessions of 40 minutes each, children were able to use biofeedback to increase the temperature of their fingertips by increasing the blood flow to their hands. As a result, their headaches went away.

ent in different people. Estrogen helps relieve some headaches but just aggravates others.

Forty female migraine sufferers were split into two groups, with 20 receiving an oral contraceptive and 20 not receiving it. Then the groups were reversed and their headaches were compared. Dr. Ryan found a definite increase in frequency of bad migraines. But, curiously, the Pill *decreased* the number of attacks in women whose migraines were normally mild. Overall, 12 patients had less migraine pain after taking the Pill, while 28 suffered more.

The most definite conclusion was that changing estrogen levels with the Pill also changes migraine patterns—for better or worse. While the Pill aggravates migraine for most sufferers, it also helps pacify some.

If your migraines repeatedly erupt at specific times during your menstrual cycle, or if they started after you began taking the Pill, your headaches might be estrogen related. If you suspect they are, ask your doctor for help with your estrogen levels.

You might also want to try supplementing your diet with magnesium. Researcher Kenneth Weaver, M.D., of the Quillen-Dishner School of Medicine at East Tennessee State University, says that magnesium therapy helped 70 percent of the 500 women he studied, stopping their migraines. Another 10 percent showed improvement. Under his direction they took 100 to 200 milligrams daily. "These patients got relief very quickly," Dr. Weaver says, adding that "the results, of course, have to be confirmed by further research."

FINDING RELIEF

For both men and women, there are several new therapies that relieve migraines. Not all are commonly used by doctors—but all of them work.

Augustus S. Rose, M.D., professor emeritus of neurology at the UCLA School of Medicine, advocates hot-and-cold showers and says that for some people they work well. He suggests that at the onset of a migraine you take a long, hot shower, then follow it with a cold shower that leaves you shivering. Often, he says, this method can actually short-circuit the impending pain.

These hot-and-cold showers are not for the elderly or those with certain chronic diseases. For these people, says Dr. Rose, crushed ice held in the mouth can sometimes accomplish the same thing as a shower.

Raising the temperature of the hands and fingers through biofeedback training, as discussed in chapter 9, also is believed to relieve migraine by easing the pressure on cerebral blood vessels. A joint study by researchers at the University of Michigan and the Scripps Clinic found that 11 migraine patients who learned the technique showed a "statistically significant and clinically therapeutic improvement" when compared with a control group.

A study of graduates of a biofeedback hand-warming class at the Menninger Foundation in Topeka, Kansas, showed that after two years the people had less intense headaches and used less medication than those who had dropped out of the class.

Another stimulating treatment for migraine is acupuncture. An Indiana University School of Medicine study showed that of 25 migraine sufferers who underwent acupuncture treatment, 68 percent were improved enough to stop medication; common migraine symptoms, including nausea, were reduced by 82 percent; and 12 people in the group felt completely well.

In a British study conducted at the National Hospital for Nervous Diseases in London, 24 of 41 patients improved after acupuncture. And a survey of acupuncture patients at the University of Alabama Medical Center concluded that the therapy may possibly release morphinelike compounds in the blood vessels, dilating them and improving oxygen supply to the tissue.

Acupressure, a similar treatment in which finger pressure is used on acupuncture points, has relieved migraine and tension headaches for hundreds of patients over a period of ten years, reports Howard D. Kurland, M.D., of Northwestern University Medical School in Chicago.

Specific types of headaches re-

Does a Greater Brain Mean Greater Pain?

If you have migraines, take heart in the fact that you are in good company: Julius Caesar, Ulysses S. Grant, Thomas Jefferson, Edgar Allan Poe, Lewis Carroll, Charles Dickens, Peter Tchaikovsky, Frederic Chopin and Charles Darwin all had migraines. But don't think having migraines makes you a genius, because there probably isn't any connection between the two. Neither is there evidence that these geniuses were better able to cope with their migraines than the average Joe. In most cases they just resorted to a grin-and-bear-it attitude, though some tried creative cures.

Ulysses S. Grant tried hot baths and mustard plasters, but soon discovered that the best medicine for his migraine problem was winning a battle with the Confederacy. And Lewis Carroll is suspected of turning his furious affliction to his own novel advantage.

In Carroll's case, medical historians have noticed a striking similarity between the bizarre scenarios and weird characters in *Alice in Wonderland* and the visual eccentricities of the "aura" phenomenon that precedes classic migraine attacks—explosions of light, feelings of vertigo or falling sensations and distorted depth, time and size perceptions. Remember Alice following the strange clock-watching White Rabbit, falling down the hole and even consuming the "drink me" potion that made her shrink? Perhaps Carroll's muse was a menacing migraine.

quire specific treatments. Most headaches seem to share one factor—stress. To assess the effects of lifestyle on a headache pattern, Dr. Diamond suggests making a careful emotional inventory. "Our patients are cautioned about trying to live up to superhuman expectations," he says. "By striving for perfection, they also induce headaches."

To put together this inventory, Dr. Diamond recommends keeping a daily record of activities—work, family, marriage, friends, whatever—along with a record of headaches, noting their severity. The purpose is to discover the emotional causes of headaches so they can be prevented in the future.

With thoughtful prevention and prompt treatment, headaches can become a thing of the past.

4

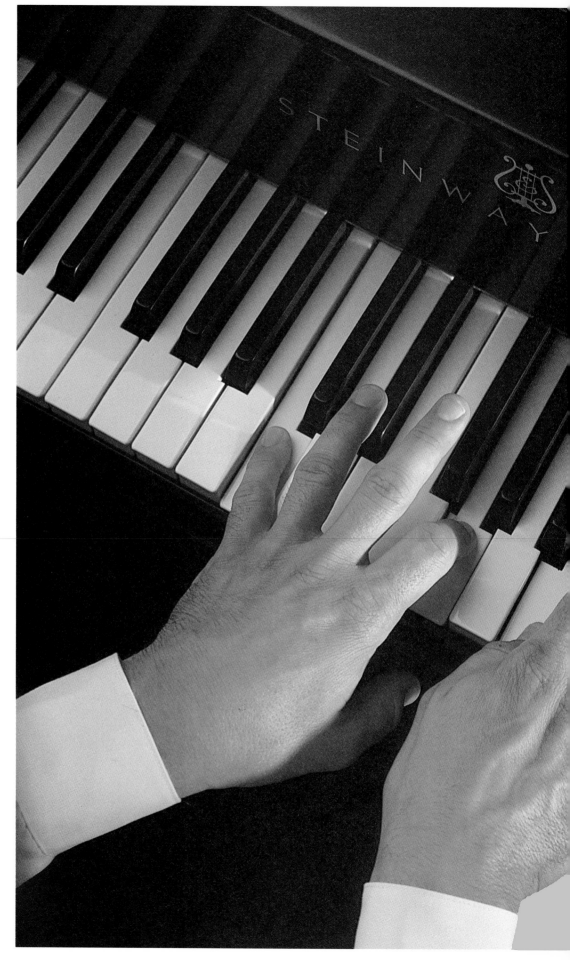

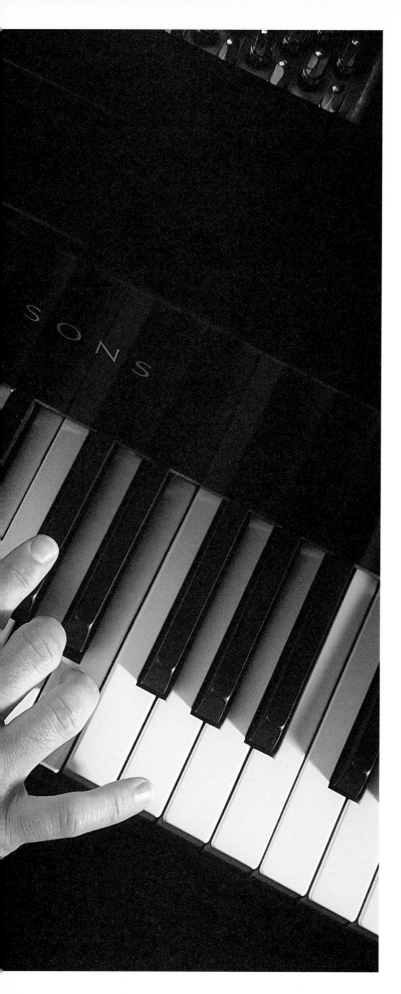

Freeing Your Bones and Joints

Here's how to relieve the pains of arthritis, gout, osteoporosis, adult rickets and TMJ disorder.

"Sixty percent of all pain complaints" are the result of bone pain (along with muscle pain caused by bone problems), says Edward J. Resnick, M.D. And he should know. He is the director of Temple University's pain control center, a last-chance stop for people who can't get rid of their pain. But if Dr. Resnick sees the hopeless, he's quick to point out that for most people with aching bones and joints, there's plenty of hope.

"This problem is almost always treatable," he says. "People who work with their doctors and take a role in their own treatment will probably never have to visit a pain control clinic."

That's great news, because bone pain can *seem* like a one-way street called misery. It's even a little painful just thinking about:

- The hot poker of arthritis pain that inflames joints and makes simple everyday movement —as well as life itself—a difficult proposition.

- Bones that become brittle or soft and weak due to insufficient calcium. Called osteoporosis and osteomalacia (*osteo-*, from the Greek, means "bone"), these problems can lead to broken bones (the kind of problem that can break your spirit, too) or muscle and bone pain.

- The long-distance pain of TMJ disorder that begins with a misaligned jaw but can end up as headaches, earaches and other pains that range from your head all the way down to your toes.

These problems have one thing in common besides bones—they're treatable. The skeleton isn't a static collection of white girders that inevitably rusts and collapses; a bone problem doesn't mean the body's architecture is ready to be condemned. Bones are a living system, and like any collection of cells they can be revitalized—and relieved of pain. Here's how.

Knuckle Cracking and Arthritis

Teachers and parents who warn that popping your knuckles will make them huge and arthritic are a little knuckleheaded. John Weber, M.D., a Philadelphia hand surgeon, explains that most arthritis of the hands shows up in finger joints and tips, not in the knuckles that are usually cracked —those at the base of the fingers. And that popping noise you hear is "definitely not bones cracking against each other." He says the sound is made when gases from the body rush into the joint to fill the space that the cracking opens.

ARTHRITIS: DOUSING THE FLAME

Arthritis is number one on the pain parade (a dubious honor). When it comes to the sheer numbers of people disabled by the 100 or so ailments grouped under the name of arthritis, other pain problems don't even come close.

Arthritis means that the joint where two bones meet is inflamed. Deep inside, your body feels like it's on fire. Every movement hurts.

What can people do when this awful pain strikes? When the first twinge pierces their hips, when a dull ache begins to gnaw at their fingers?

If they're like Marcella Cokkinis, they can say thanks—thanks for the pain.

"I APPRECIATE THE PAIN"

"I never thought the day would come when I would hear myself say, 'I appreciate pain,'" Marcella admits. But the active mother of two children realizes that "had I not felt the pain, the arthritis would have silently and secretly crept up on me until all of a sudden I might have found myself an invalid for no apparent reason. The pain was a warning sign, and I'm grateful."

You don't hear many people being grateful for rheumatoid arthritis. Rheumatoid arthritis is a disease that damages and inflames the tissues around the joints. It's usually chronic. There is no cure.

It can attack and inflame any area of the body—skin, muscles, blood vessels—in addition to the joints. Unlike the more common osteoarthritis, it's not the result of years of wear and tear or of an old injury, and it doesn't stay limited to just a few joints. It spreads its pain throughout the entire body.

Yet Marcella Cokkinis now hikes in the High Sierras and the Grand Canyon. She plays soccer on a women's team. She'll always have rheumatoid arthritis—but she knows how to make it reasonably pain free.

Her positive attitude—seeing her pain as a warning signal instead of an unbeatable enemy—allowed her

to get an early start on controlling that pain. Unfortunately, most people wait an average of four years after their first symptoms appear before they seek treatment.

Four years! Imagine what would happen to your car if you let a strange noise under the hood go unchecked for that long! With arthritis, instead of a damaged engine, the result can be damaged joints.

In either case, preventive maintenance is the key to avoiding costly repairs. With cars, you listen for gremlins under the hood or watch for smoke from the tailpipe. With arthritis, you want to be on the lookout for these early warning signs:

- Swelling in one or more joints.
- Early morning stiffness.
- Constant or recurring pain or tenderness in a joint.
- Inability to move a joint or any part of your body as you used to.
- Warmth or redness in a joint.
- Unexpected weight loss, fever or weakness combined with joint pain.

If you have two or more of these symptoms, you should see a doctor—preferably an arthritis specialist (a rheumatologist)—for diagnosis and proper treatment.

In addition to the help your doctor gives you, there are lots of things you can do on your own. A few sensible acts of prevention now, explains Dr. Resnick, can keep the pain of arthritis at bay for the rest of your life.

THE PAIN-RELIEF DIET

Most important, he feels, is keeping your weight down. (Being just 10 percent overweight puts you at a higher risk of *developing* arthritis.) The last thing a joint that's already under stress needs is more weight to support. "A good low-fat diet to lose weight, combined with an exercise program to keep the pounds off, can alleviate 75 percent of the pain and other symptoms in arthritis patients," says Art Mollen, D.O., founder and director of the Southwest Health Institute in Phoenix, Arizona.

Low fat may mean low pain for

Exercise against Arthritis

These exercises are excellent drug-free ways to limit the pain of arthritis and increase your range of motion. Always remember to warm up slowly with gentle stretching before exercising. And don't exercise when your joints are really hot and painful. As a general rule, move the joint as far as it will go comfortably and then take it a little further, just past that first sign of pain. Repeat each exercise at least 3 times to start and work up to 10 repetitions, 2 to 4 times a day. Start slow and easy. If pain persists for more than 2 hours following exercise, you need to cut back. But don't quit. Remember that for maximum pain relief you must move each joint through its full range of motion every day.

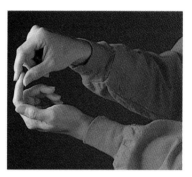

Fingers

If your fingers are stiff, gently curl the very tip of your finger toward the palm (use the opposite hand to guide it if necessary). Then bend the middle part inward, followed by the knuckle. If your fingers are curled up to begin with, perform the same exercise in reverse.

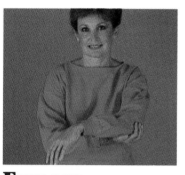

Shoulders

Here's a good way to ease a painful shoulder. Stand or sit, then lean slightly forward. Let your arms hang in front of you, but keep them straight. Make little circling motions with your arms, gradually increasing the size of the circles.

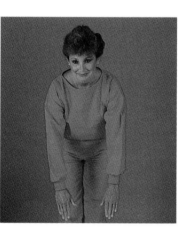

Forearm

If it is painful to turn a doorknob, try this: Rest your arm on a table with the palm down. Slowly rotate your arm so that the palm faces up. If you have to use your other arm to help, use it to move the forearm, not the hand itself.

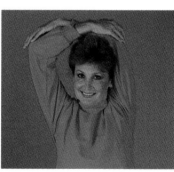

The Shoulder Cradle

Another cure for a sore shoulder: Hold your elbow with the opposite hand and slowly raise it above your head. You can even rest the arm on top of your head as you coax it back a little further. If this is difficult, you can lie down to do the exercise.

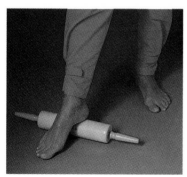

Feet

Here's a good roll for those hot dogs. Put a round dowel, like a broomstick or a rolling pin, on the floor. Then place the arch of your foot on top and slowly roll it back and forth.

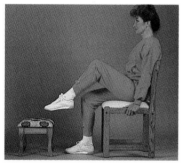

Knees

Too much sitting can make your knee ligaments tight and painful. Relax them by sitting in a chair with your foot up on another chair or a high footstool. Bend your knee up and then straighten it out again. If this exercise gets too easy, stay in the same position and lean forward carefully while keeping your back nice and straight to stretch your hamstring muscles.

reasons other than weight loss. Two researchers at Wayne State University in Detroit have found that the painful swelling and stiffness of rheumatoid arthritis appears to be aggravated by fatty foods and can be dramatically reduced by a low-fat diet. In two patients with rheumatoid arthritis, stiffness and swelling in their joints went away within days after they went on a low-calorie, low-fat diet—and they remained symptom free for 9 to 14 months. However, within 24 to 48 hours of eating fatty foods, the researchers report, the stiffness returned.

Though they caution that the experimental group tested to date is a small one (it included 6 arthritis patients in all), the researchers write in *Clinical Research* that it's possible that "dietary fats in amounts normally eaten in the American diet cause the inflammatory joint changes seen in rheumatoid arthritis."

THE RIGHT MOVES

Mary P. Schatz, M.D., considers exercise essential to ending the pain of arthritis. The Nashville, Tennessee, physician and yoga instructor points out that only exercise can restore health to the area where arthritis strikes: the cartilage.

The cartilage is the "shock absorber" that sits on the ends of the bones where they meet. It's surrounded by fluid (called synovial fluid) that sends nutrients into the cartilage and removes waste.

Without movement, the joint begins to starve and waste products are trapped. The arthritis gets worse, pain is increased, and range of motion becomes even more limited.

With movement, oxygen and nutrients work their way in, waste is removed, and swelling and pain are reduced.

Besides "feeding" the joint itself, exercise increases the strength and flexibility of the muscles and ligaments surrounding the joints. When strength increases, pain decreases. But many arthritis patients neglect exercise. That's a big mistake, according to George Ehrlich, M.D., a nationally recognized arthritis specialist who is currently vice president for anti-inflammatory drugs for Ciba-Geigy Pharmaceutical Corporation.

"Patients who exercise manage their arthritis very well—and aren't held back by it in the least," he says—if they exercise correctly.

(continued on page 44)

Copper Bracelets: Fad or Fact?

The Arthritis Foundation classifies copper bracelets as "unproven remedies," along with sitting in old uranium mines and covering yourself with cow manure twice a day. But copper makes more sense than cow manure, and not just for aesthetic reasons. According to John R. J. Sorenson, Ph.D., of the University of Arkansas Medical School, a deficiency of copper is known to cause pain in connective tissue and abnormalities in the bones and joints. He says a lack of copper can also weaken the immune system and make inflammation worse.

But when you get enough, copper interacts with aspirin to act as an anti-inflammatory. Enzymes that depend on copper aid in the repair of inflamed body tissues, as well.

So there's a case for copper. But why in bracelets and not in supplements? Copper poisoning is why. Too much can make you sick and hurt your kidneys, liver and brain.

You don't have these problems with bracelets. But you might have benefits. Australian physicians compared the effects of copper bracelets to aluminum fakes that looked the same as copper. The arthritis patients wearing the real ones felt less pain than the control group wearing the fakes.

The real bracelets also lost a measurable amount of copper, which was absorbed through the skin.

The Arthritis Foundation worries that people who try unproven remedies like the bracelets will neglect other therapies and expect a miracle cure. Meanwhile, their condition could get worse, and even result in joint damage.

Allay their fears—and yours. Wear any kind of jewelry you like, but keep up with your other treatments.

Betty Jane Gregor
East Greenville, Pa.
Rheumatoid Arthritis

B.J. fights her arthritis with fervor. Her swollen hands and fingers don't stop her from painting and writing. Her ankles and wrists are weak, but using her forearms to push a raised, padded chair on wheels in front of her allows her to get around the house just fine. If there's something she can't do, she and her husband devise gadgets or rearrange things until she can. Twenty-one years ago, the doctor who finally diagnosed the cause of the intense pains in her hands told her and her husband William to "psych themselves up for a wheelchair, because she'll be in one by Christmas." She now realizes he was challenging her to prove him wrong. And she did. But it wasn't always easy.

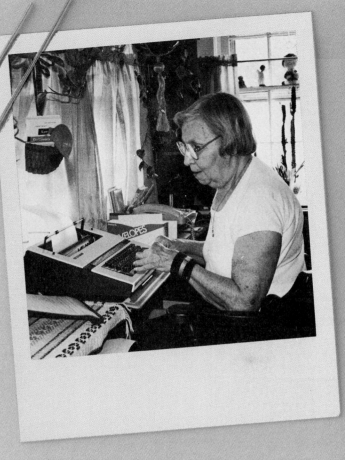

"I once spent 8 months without ever leaving the house," she says, talking about the "4 years of hell" during which she could only sleep for about 15 minutes at a time "because the pain was so constant." The turning point came when she realized that she had begun to just sit in a chair 12 hours a day for days at a time. She knew that, unless things changed, this was going to be her life from then on.

She began by establishing her own identity and interests. She coined the name B.J. for herself and began painting. She claims to be the least talented person in the world, but the serene landscapes that hang in her perfectly kept home deny that. "You have to learn to live outside of yourself and then you can learn to live with the pain," she explains.

Now she helps others live with theirs. Following an intensive training program, she became "the token arthritic" for the Arthritis Foundation's local self-help course.

"I'm here so that you don't have to go through the years of trial and error that I did," she tells members of the group during their first meeting. As the weeks progress she will try to draw them out—get them to talk about their problems, encourage them to exercise, and demand that they "rest without feeling ashamed about it."

"Arthritis is a very personal thing," she stresses. "A support group like this lets them know that there are other people who are hurting; that they're not alone. It takes people a while to realize that the arthritis is simply not going to go away. But once they realize that they *can* keep it from getting worse, they're on their way."

B.J. uses her positive attitude and example to convey an important message. "You can prevent a lot of the pain and deformity," she tells the group, "but it's 80 percent you and only 20 percent your doctor."

41

Help Yourself to Less Pain

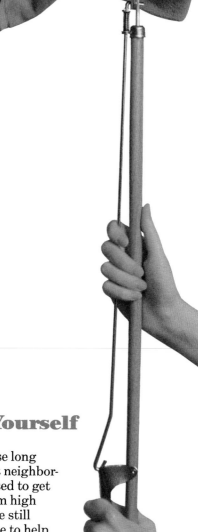

Taking the pain out of arthritis requires more than proper exercise, medication and getting enough rest. It also means thinking of ways to make everyday activities easier and more efficient. Often just a slight modification in the way you do things can make the difference. Here are some nifty devices that you might want to try to make life easier. You can buy some at the store, but you'll want to ask a friend or a local handyman for help in making the others.

Hold Tight

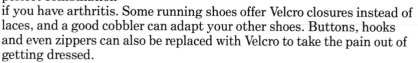

The space-age material Velcro holds fast when you press the two pieces together, yet pulls apart easily with a light touch—a perfect combination if you have arthritis. Some running shoes offer Velcro closures instead of laces, and a good cobbler can adapt your other shoes. Buttons, hooks and even zippers can also be replaced with Velcro to take the pain out of getting dressed.

Extend Yourself

Remember those long "grabbers" that neighborhood grocers used to get items down from high shelves? They're still around. Buy one to help you get things down from high places or up off the floor.

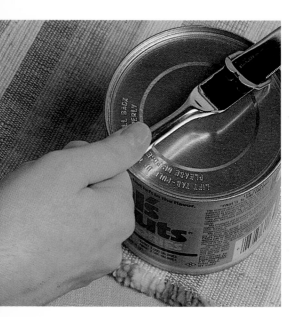

Can Do

Flip-top cans flip you out? Slide the blade of a butter knife through the tab, then press down on the handle with your palm.

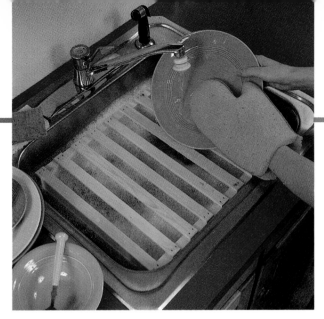

Washing Dishes

Buy a sponge mitt to wash dishes. A wooden rack made of lattice board in the sink will keep you from having to reach down low to get to the dishes.

Turning Doorknobs

Nobody can get a good grip on those smooth, round doorknobs. You can buy a large rubber lever that fits over top or, better still, have the whole knob replaced with a lever or "French doorknob" from the hardware store.

Getting a Grip on Things

Slide foam hair curlers over the handles of hair brushes and rattail combs, silverware, pens and pencils —anything small and round that needs a built-up grip. For larger troublesome items, glue bicycle handlebar grips onto their handles for a grip you just can't lose.

Don't Touch That Dial

Any good-sized block of wood is all you need to regain control over your TV set, air conditioner, washer, dryer or other large appliance. Have a deep slot carved in one end and you'll have all the leverage you need to turn control knobs.

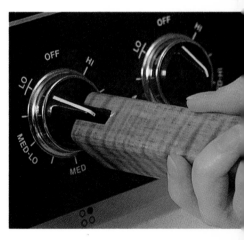

Card Holder

A nice flat piece of wood with ¼-inch slots cut into it is great for holding cards. (But it won't help if you draw on an inside straight.)

HOW TO EXERCISE SAFELY

Any exercise-induced pain that lasts longer than 2 hours warns you that you pushed your joints too far, too fast. If you have this sort of pain, talk to your physical therapist about ways to take it a little easier next time. Be patient. It may take a while to put together the program that suits you best, but don't give up.

And exercise is an everyday requirement. Even when joints are stiff and achy, you *still* must move them through their full range of motion twice a day, but gently and easily.

Here are some tips that will make exercising an easier experience.

- Don't fight morning stiffness. Exercise during the part of the day when you feel your best (usually midafternoon).
- *Really* warm up. Take a hot bath or shower before you stretch. It'll relax joints and muscles and relieve pain.
- Learn some good warm-up techniques such as gentle stretching and use them before exercising.
- Begin exercises with small, pain-free movements and gradually work up to the real thing.
- Begin at a comfortable level and gradually increase the number of repetitions. Progress slowly to avoid unnecessary pain.
- Do your exercises with a slow, steady rhythm. Give your muscles 10 to 15 seconds to relax between repetitions. This rhythm should make the program more effective and enjoyable.
- Breathe deeply and rhythmically. Don't hold your breath. Ask your doctor or physical therapist to help you with deep breathing exercises.
- Don't take extra medication thinking that it will help you exercise more with less pain. Excessive pain is one sure warning that you're doing too much. Masking the pain could lead you to damage the joints.
- Move each joint as far as it will go comfortably and then coax it a little further—just past the first twinge of pain.
- Stretching exercises should be repeated three to ten times each, two to four times a day, depending on the pain.
- In order for your pain not to worsen, you must move every joint in your body through its full range of motion—duplicating all the movements that a healthy joint can normally perform—twice a day. This includes the joints you may be "protecting" because they hurt.

The exercises on page 39 are range-of-motion, or stretching, exercises. A complete program will also include strengthening exercises—such as isometrics—to lend more stability to the joints themselves, and endurance exercises like swimming or walking.

For the best results, a balance must be struck between exercise and rest. In this case, "rest" means quiet time—we're not talking about sewing or light housework. You're entitled to this quiet time every day. Avoiding fatigue allows you to exercise correctly when the time comes.

A HOT IDEA

Exercise isn't the only therapy you can warm up to. "Some of the things that really work best against arthritis pain involve careful application of heat. A warm bath or shower—not too hot!—can be very helpful," says Dr. Ehrlich.

When applied by someone your doctor recommends, "paraffin baths can be very good for arthritis in the hands. Heat relaxes the area to relieve the pain," explains Dr. Ehrlich.

On the other hand, an ice pack—or even a bag of frozen vegetables—will help cool acute pain by reducing swelling and inflammation. "Cold is a temporary analgesic for acute—not chronic—pain," says Dr. Ehrlich.

USING DRUGS SAFELY

When it comes to drugs, Dr. Ehrlich feels that aspirin and the other nonsteroidal anti-inflammatory drugs (NSAIDs)—including ibuprofen, naproxen and indomethacin—are effective when taken in the correct dose. By reducing the inflammation, they get rid of the pain.

Nevertheless, a rheumatologist will generally start with aspirin, although the doses used to control the pain of arthritis (16 to 20 regular tablets a day for the inflammation that accompanies rheumatoid arthritis; 12 a day for osteoarthritis) can cause serious stomach irritation if you don't take precautions.

To limit these effects, take the aspirin with food at each meal and at bedtime. Eat a bit, take the aspirin and then finish eating. Or take the aspirin with a glass of milk.

THE "EXQUISITE" PAIN OF GOUT

"The victim goes to bed and sleeps in good health. About two o'clock in the morning he is awakened by a severe pain in the great toe; more rarely in the heel, ankle or instep. This pain is like that of a dislocation, and yet the parts feel as if cold water were poured over them.

"Then follow chills and shivers and a little fever. The pain, which was at first moderate, becomes more intense. . . . Now it is a violent stretching and tearing of the ligaments . . . a gnawing pain . . . a pressure and tightening."

The part "affected cannot bear the weight of bedclothes nor the jar of a person walking in the room. The night is passed in torture, sleeplessness, turning of the part affected and perpetual change of posture; the tossing about of the body being as incessant as the pain of the tortured joint, and being worse as the fit comes on."

Not much has changed in the 300 years since Sir Thomas Sydenham—"the English Hippocrates" and founder of clinical medicine—penned this famous description of a typical first attack of the gout.

What causes this pain? Needle-sharp crystals of uric acid that slowly build up and inflame a single joint, usually below the waist but some-times in the shoulders, spine or jaw.

At least half of all first attacks strike the big toe, with the pain arriving as a middle-of-the-night wake-up call that feels as though it were delivered with a sledgehammer. "Exquisitely painful" is how the standard *Textbook of Rheumatology* describes this form of arthritis.

Some victims feel short twinges of pain prior to the attack and simply "walk them off." But for most the pain strikes with explosive suddenness—the joint becomes red and inflamed, swelling to extreme tenderness.

Replacement Parts for Painful Joints

Hips that have lost their swivel, knees that can't kneel and fingers that fail to flex are the kinds of painful problems that make arthritis sufferers wish they could just trade in their old, damaged joints for new ones.

That wish has become reality. The ability to replace damaged joints with man-made materials is medical fact, not science fiction—and it offers pain relief at levels previously undreamed of.

"The best candidate is someone with osteoarthritis of the hip or knee, because the disease is limited to the joint that's going to be replaced," says Frederic C. McDuffie, M.D., senior vice-president of medical affairs for The Arthritis Foundation.

People with rheumatoid arthritis also experience great pain relief when those same worn-out parts are replaced with space-age metal and plastic components, but the procedure doesn't help relieve pain in their other joints.

In either case, hip and knee replacements "restore much of the range of motion that was lost, and relieve 95 percent or more of the pain in the affected area," says Dr. McDuffie.

Hands, unfortunately, are a different matter. Because they are so small in comparison to hips or knees and have such tiny muscles, replacement of finger joints "doesn't provide the kind of improvement in function that you see with hips. But it does improve the appearance of the hand dramatically, and it's a great operation for pain relief."

The pain can last anywhere from a few hours to several weeks before subsiding. While it may never return, the next attack for most gout victims is only six months to two years away.

Most victims are male, about age 50. They may inherit the tendency toward gout, or it may be the result of taking diuretic medications for control of high blood pressure, explains Charles D. Tourtellotte, M.D., professor of medicine and chief of rheumatology at Temple University Hospital.

Whatever the cause, when you wake up in the middle of the night with a big toe that is about to explode, you want relief—fast. What should you do?

BLUNTING THE NEEDLES

Several medications are extremely effective at putting out the fire, says John B. Winfield, M.D., chief of the division of rheumatology at the University of North Carolina School of Medicine. These include certain nonsteroidal anti-inflammatory drugs. Dr. Winfield explains that both indomethacin and ibuprofen are "very effective in treating acute gout."

Aspirin, which is so effective in treating other arthritis, should not be used in gout because it, paradoxically, may increase the risk of attacks. The reason for this is that aspirin may raise the level of uric acid in the blood.

But *don't* waste time. The sooner you start taking a NSAID the better your recovery will be, according to the *Textbook of Rheumatology.* The book also suggests you take a NSAID at the first twinge of an attack. If you act quickly enough, a small dose may be all you need.

But rather than waiting until the next attack strikes, do the following to prevent pain in the future:

Lose Weight. Dr. Tourtellotte feels that obese people "have a metabolic derangement that causes them to retain uric acid." But don't go on a crash diet, since many doctors say it may also cause you to retain the acid, causing an attack.

Cut Back on Alcohol. Dr. Tourtellotte warns that "alcohol itself will incite acute gout attacks." Mostly we're talking about chronic alcohol use, but beer, heavy wines and champagnes actually seem to deserve their historical connection as the cause of the elevated aching toe. So be moderate.

Limit Purine-Rich Foods. People with gout either produce too much uric acid to begin with or produce the right amount but don't get rid of it normally. When enough of it hangs around, it's lured to a single joint and the result is a gout attack. Purines (the "parent" compound of uric acids) in the diet can aggravate uric acid problems. Eating a low-purine diet will lower the body's uric acid levels. So limit your intake of the following purine-rich foods: anchovies, artichokes, bacon, codfish, goose, haddock, herring, kidneys, liver, mackerel, mussels, mutton, salmon, sardines, scallops, smelt, sweetbreads, trout, turkey, veal, venison and yeast.

"Most meats are very high in purines," notes Dr. Tourtellote, "so a low-purine diet would be mainly a vegetarian diet."

THE CASE OF THE VANISHING SKELETON

Osteoporosis. There's usually no warning, except for possible lower back pain. This "silent disease" often says its first hello with a broken bone. A bone that has been "thinning" —losing its actual substance as hormonal changes allow the calcium to drift out of a woman's body following menopause.

An orthopedic specialist will tend to the fracture and prescribe medication to ease the pain as the bone and surrounding tissues heal. In addition, Morris Notelovitz, M.D., coauthor of *Stand Tall! The Informed Woman's Guide to Preventing Osteoporosis,* "would definitely also give . . . estrogen."

Dr. Notelovitz feels that the use of estrogen immediately after a fracture will serve to actually reduce the pain by stopping the tiny microfractures that would otherwise continue to appear in the bones as the osteoporosis progresses.

Without the formation of new

microfractures, the broken bone can heal more cleanly and quickly. Stopping these tiny fractures also reduces the risk of major breaks, both while the current fracture is healing and afterward.

If you want to completely avoid the pain and disfigurement that accompany osteoporosis, Dr. Notelovitz suggests you get started early in life with a program designed to build up bone strength. He says age 25 isn't too early for women to begin exercising to build bone mass and to make sure they get enough calcium and vitamin D.

ADULT RICKETS

It begins with fatigue and aching bones. Soon the pain in the bones becomes severe. Extreme muscle weakness sets in. If the condition is left untreated, the patient becomes bedridden, with tiny fractures all through the body.

Bones that once were strong, bracing structures like the steel girders of a skyscraper now resemble the ancient wooden beams of an old, ready-to-collapse building.

The condition: osteomalacia, also known as adult rickets. The cause: not enough vitamin D. While calcium prevents the roof from crashing in, your bones need vitamin D to properly absorb that mineral. You get D free of charge from sunlight and from foods like herring, mackerel, sardines, salmon, tuna, swordfish and shrimp. Fish-liver oils are also high in the vitamin. And the best way to get vitamin D and calcium together is from milk.

Until recently most doctors thought that a vitamin D deficiency was rare in adults. Unfortunately, that's not so. Some elderly people don't drink milk, eat fish, take cod-liver oil or get much sun. So they get little vitamin D. Their bodies still get calcium, however—by stealing it from their very skeletons. The result is pain and broken bones.

"As many as 30 to 40 percent of all hip fracture patients in the U.S. have osteomalacia," estimates Samuel H. Doppelt, M.D., of Harvard Medical School. Uriel S. Barzel, M.D.,

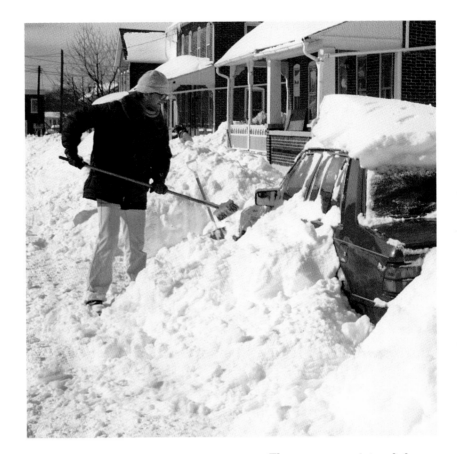

professor of medicine at Albert Einstein Medical College in New York City feels that the condition is much more common than was generally believed and "that it should be routinely considered in all older patients with vague complaints of pain and weakness."

Dr. Barzel treats his osteomalacia patients with a regimen of 1,500 milligrams a day of calcium, plus large amounts of vitamin D (the Recommended Dietary Allowance is 400 I.U. of vitamin D a day. Always check with your doctor before taking more than this). Within two weeks of starting these treatments, his patients feel stronger. After a few months, their bones are back up to snuff, the pain is gone, and the vitamin D supplementation is reduced to 400 I.U. a day.

TMJ DISORDER:
IT'S ALL IN YOUR HEAD

Temporomandibular joint (TMJ) disorder can mimic a host of painful problems from head to toe.

The young man pictured above may be putting his back into his work, but the cold weather is preventing him from putting any sunshine onto his back— and that's the part of the body that's best at absorbing the solar rays that turn cholesterol into vitamin D. In the summer, 15 or 20 minutes a day is all the sunshine that light-pigmented people need to meet their requirement for D. But it's not as easy to use solar energy to manufacture this essential pain preventer in the wintertime, when the sun is much lower in the sky, says Uriel S. Barzel, M.D., professor of medicine at Albert Einstein Medical College in New York City. He also points out that passing through glass robs sunshine of its powers to create vitamin D, so don't expect to meet your quota by sitting near a window. Instead, Dr. Barzel says that, in the winter, older people must make sure that they take vitamin D in supplement form to prevent the eventual pain of osteomalacia.

Symptoms That Signal TMJ

Doctors call TMJ (temporomandibular joint) disorder the great impostor, because its symptoms mimic many *other* problems. Maybe you haven't thought of TMJ as the cause of your pain. If you have any of the following symptoms, maybe you should.

- Face and neck pain
- Migraine headaches
- Backache
- Sinus trouble
- Hearing loss
- Earache
- Ringing in the ears
- Difficulty in swallowing
- Burning tongue
- Dizziness
- Fatigue
- Poor coordination
- Stiff neck
- Sore shoulders
- Numbness in limbs
- Cold hands
- Tingling sensation
- Limited motion in arms and legs

Deborah Turner's bout with this "great impostor" began with an earache. Even though there was no infection, her doctor gave her a prescription for antibiotics and sent her on her way.

Then came the headaches. "My entire head would pound and throb so badly I'd be incapacitated," she explains. Aspirin helped at first, but soon even large doses had no effect.

She started to feel a toothache whenever she ate hard foods. The ache soon became a constant, throbbing pain. X rays showed no problem, but her dentist started drilling anyway, to "even up" her teeth.

The mystery pain moved on. Now it ruled from her jaw down her shoulder and into her arms and fingers. Her entire right side above the waist became painful to the touch. She thought for sure she had a serious back problem.

Finally, some of the doctors and dentists she saw started blaming her jaw. Even though the worst pain was in her neck and shoulder blades, the real villain had finally been uncovered in her head.

Where had it all started? Was it with the tooth a dentist had pulled "to ease crowding" in her mouth? The sudden jolt she had received in a car crash? The smack in the head when the boat she was sailing overturned? The wisdom teeth that were pulled?

All are possibilities. But whatever the cause, her jaw was out of alignment and sending waves of pain throughout her body.

Many people call Deborah Turner's problem TMJ, which stands for—take a deep breath—temporomandibular joint. You can feel yours right now by placing your fingers on your jaw in front of your ears. It will move when you open and close your mouth.

You can feel the effects of that same joint all the way up to your temples—and higher. Its movements cover a wide area and can cause an even wider variety of problems (see "Symptoms That Signal TMJ").

Misalignment of this essential joint—which is located near the major arteries and veins running to the brain—often goes undetected because much of the pain it causes is "referred" to other areas of the body. Physicians treating a numb arm, for instance, rarely look to the jaw as a possible cause.

BE SKEPTICAL, BE SAFE

Some health professionals, however, have a tendency to lean too far in the other direction. They're aware that the TMJ can play a role in mysterious pains and they go overboard, blaming it for everything that is wrong with a person.

"Just because someone's jaw hurts doesn't mean they have a TMJ problem," explains S. Gary Cohen, D.M.D., of the University of Pennsylvania Hospital's TMJ clinic. "The same kind of pain caused by TMJ could be the result of a muscular problem or an infection. An ear infection, especially, will cause exactly the same type of pains in the ear and face."

So, like Debbie Turner, you could wind up being treated for something other than your TMJ problem. Or you could be treated for TMJ disorder when you *really* only have an ear infection. In either case, the end result is a lot of time wasted with misdiagnosis and a lot of inappropriate treatment before you finally find relief from the pain.

"Many people have had the problem for years and have seen many types of health professionals before they get to our program," explains Dr. Cohen. "Unfortunately, by the time they *do* get here, most have become chronic pain sufferers. They've seen at least 4 health professionals previously—doctors, dentists, physical therapists, acupuncturists—and some have seen as many as 20!"

Headaches are often a clue to a TMJ problem. Lawrence A. Funt, D.D.S., director of the Cranio-Facial Pain Center in Bethesda, Maryland, urges all health professionals to check for TMJ disorder by asking their headache patients if they also have a dull ache on one side of their jaw, tenderness, clicking, locking or pain on chewing.

A history of allergies or other respiratory problems should also be a clue, says Dr. Funt. He feels that people with those conditions may develop the bad habit of breathing through the mouth instead of the nose. "Open-mouth breathing," Dr. Funt explains, "puts an inordinate strain on the muscles surrounding the jaws, in the throat and in the neck and shoulders."

Those strains on the neck and shoulder muscles are the cause of the "referred pain" of TMJ disorder that can be felt almost anywhere in the body. "People with pain in the neck and shoulders will hold themselves poorly," explains Dr. Cohen, "causing soreness and tenderness in other parts of the body that may seem more painful than the jaw itself."

IS IT OR ISN'T IT TMJ?

Before you blame TMJ disorder for your pain, be sure you meet the criteria. Here are some ways to rule yourself in or out of the TMJ club:

"It *can't* be TMJ," explains Dr. Cohen, "if the patient has full range of motion and no tenderness in the jaw. You *don't* have TMJ disorder if you can open your jaw and put in three fingers (one on top of the other) without it hurting. Or if you can turn your head left and right or eat without pain."

Now, here's a test to see if you are at risk of having or developing a TMJ problem. Irwin Smigel, D.D.S., author of *Dental Health, Dental Beauty,* says to place your little fingers in your ears and press them forward, then open and close your jaws. If you hear a clicking sound in either ear, it means things are not quite centered in your jaw.

This is the easiest TMJ symptom to spot—but don't panic if you hear a click. It may never graduate to full-fledged pain. "On the other hand," warns Dr. Smigel, "it is an alerting signal to possible sudden pain in the future."

GET IT RIGHT THE FIRST TIME

If you do suspect TMJ is causing your pain, walk—do *not* run—to a dentist for treatment. And take your skepticism along with you. The wrong approach to your problem could make it much, much worse.

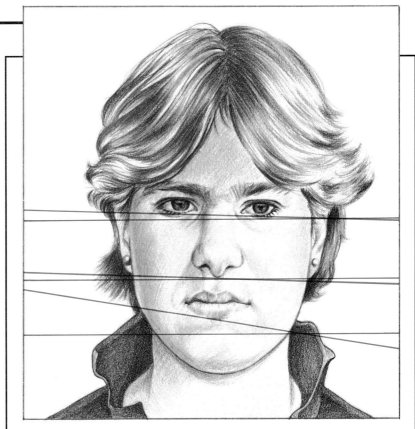

The Subtle Signs of TMJ Disorder

What do this young woman's features have in common with the average checkbook?

Neither one is balanced. One of the primary symptoms of a TMJ problem is that a person will appear lopsided if you look very carefully.

This subtle misalignment will be most obvious in the facial area, with what professionals refer to as "feature imbalance." As in the illustration, one eye may seem to be higher, and even slightly larger, than the other; the bottoms of the ears may not be level; and the jaw line may be uneven. Often the lips on the side of the affected joint will be turned up.

In fact, that entire half of the body may be off-center. The shoulder, breast hip and leg will appear to be lower.

A full-length mirror will help confirm the problem. Look at yourself carefully and, if you have any aches or pains that seem confined to one side, check that side for misalignment.

Fortunately, as you work to correct the TMJ problem, your face, posture and body parts may follow your jaw as it's coaxed back into proper alignment.

Car Crash? Think Jawlash

Been in a car accident lately? Have any aches and pains that the doctors can't chase away? Are they telling you, "It's all in your head"?

Maybe they're right—and maybe you should see a dentist who works with TMJ (temporomandibular joint) disorder patients. "Most people don't realize that the jaw is connected to the neck and receives the same kind of shock when you're in an accident," explains Harold Ravins, D.D.S., of Los Angeles. The violent motion that twists necks out of shape can do the same to a jaw by knocking it out of alignment. So brush after every meal—and maybe see a dentist after every brush with disaster.

Surgery is often presented as a first option. Other dentists may want to do lots of drilling, filling and even pulling of teeth. Dr. Cohen feels that such treatments are extremely inappropriate early in the game, and that people in pain should get another opinion.

"A good TMJ practitioner will always start with the most conservative and reversible treatments," assures Dr. Cohen. On the other hand, "the *wrong* kind of treatment generally costs around $2,500 and is performed by someone who doesn't spend much time with the patient but makes extravagant promises and assures you he has *never* had a failure."

So how can you tell if your mouth is in good hands?

"You want to start with someone who will take a really good medical history," explains Dr. Cohen. "They should ask you about *everything* that could affect the actual complaint: Have you had any recent trauma (like a fall or a car accident)—say, within the last year? What medications are you taking? What makes the pain worse? What makes it go away?

"You want to rule out as many possibilities as you can—if the pain is part of a rheumatoid arthritis problem, for instance, it may disappear with standard arthritis treatments. There may be no need for *any* kind of work on the jaw itself," he notes. "A traumatic event or injury needs to be investigated. Has the patient gotten whiplash in an auto accident? Have they been mugged? Even a long dental visit can be the cause."

A long dental visit?

"Sure," says Dr. Cohen. "Many dentists can actually create a problem far worse than the one they correct by doing too much work in one sitting and keeping the jaw frozen open for hours at a time. At our hospital we call it the business person's special: 12 years of dental work done in one 6-hour sitting."

STEP ONE: END THE PAIN

Following a good examination that lays the blame for the pain squarely on the jaw, Dr. Cohen and his associates go to work. "The first step is to get the patient out of pain," he explains. "Then you get them back into shape."

For initial pain control, Dr. Cohen uses a NSAID to relieve the pain by reducing the inflammation. NSAIDs include common aspirin as well as other drugs like ibuprofen (available over the counter) and naproxen (available by prescription only).

Application of moist heat to the affected area also relieves pain. So do exercises to ease jaw movement that you can do at home between visits.

"If the patient doesn't feel any better after two to four weeks, I like to get an appliance in," says Dr. Cohen. He's not talking about a refrigerator or a dishwasher—this "appliance" is a small piece of metal and acrylic that is fitted and inserted into the mouth to gently coax the jaw into a more tolerable position over a period of time.

"It's dental physical therapy," explains Harold Ravins, D.D.S., of Los Angeles. He has had great success in banishing pain with these appliances, each of which is specially designed and fitted according to a patient's individual needs.

"We'll place a testing appliance in the mouth to see if head and neck mobility improves, and patients notice the difference instantly," Dr. Ravins has found.

Some appliances need to be worn 24 hours a day and others only while the patient is asleep. "Nighttime is the best time for wearing an appliance, especially if you clench your teeth while you're asleep," explains Dr. Cohen.

A lifetime of clenching can knock the jaw out of line just as well as a left hook or a car accident. To treat this component of the problem, we have to get back into the ring with our old enemy, stress.

Dr. Smigel explains that "people who clench (their teeth) under frequent stress may put jaw, head, neck, shoulder and back muscles in high tension for hours rather than minutes. . . . Muscles weaken under this constant strain and may eventually go into spasm.

"Emotional stress," concludes Dr. Smigel, "unquestionably makes a major contribution to the TMJ syndrome."

Carolyn Kugel
New Castle, Del.
TMJ Disorder

The doctors talked about pinched nerves, sciatica, damaged disks. They decided she was unhappy at home, that she had a bad sex life.

Toward the end of her 20-year battle with a headache that never went away and "a constant, burning pain" in her lower back, neck and shoulder, Carolyn Kugel was convinced that she must have a brain tumor.

"The right side of my face would distort so badly, it looked like it was melting," she remembers. "When the headaches were at their worst, you could actually feel the pulsing throb on the right side of my head." The pain would radiate from the neck down, all along her right side. She would lose all the feeling and strength in her fingers.

Here was a high school English teacher who couldn't hold a piece of chalk. A mother with 2 young children who woke up with a headache every day. A wife whose husband was getting very tired of hearing her complain when he couldn't see broken bones or anything else that he could identify with "real" pain.

But someone finally began to figure it out. It happened when a family dentist who was treating her son for clenched teeth noticed that *she* was the clenching champ of all time. He told her to wear a brace at night to protect the teeth. She broke 3 of the braces. "This is not supposed to be happening," he remarked.

She visited an old friend, an oral pathologist in Texas. He saw that her whole face was "out of whack," and informed her that she had what has been dubbed the disease of the 1980s—TMJ disorder.

She started seeing a TMJ disorder specialist closer to home. He prescribed exercises and made an appliance that pulled the bottom of her jaw forward and to the left.

Slowly, over a period of months, the pains in her body disappeared. The headaches that had accompanied every moment of every day now appeared every other week or so. The "dowager's hump" she had begun to develop because of the pain in her back disappeared. She felt as though she "grew an inch."

People noticed the difference—in her face, in the shape of her mouth. She can smile now, and eat apples without having to carve them up into tiny pieces.

She still has a way to go, but the worst is over. "Even though everything isn't perfect yet, it just doesn't hurt anymore. I don't have to be numb anymore," she says.

51

5

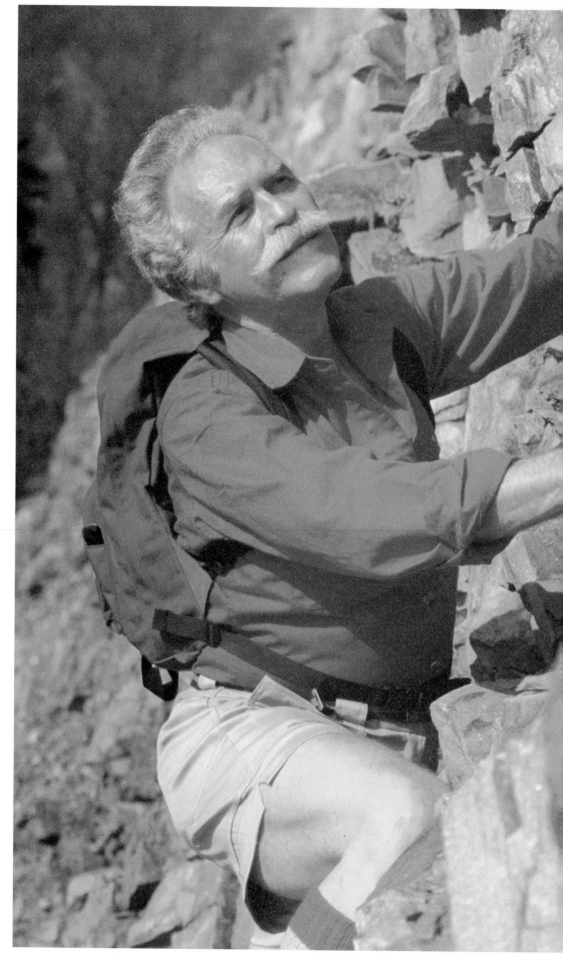

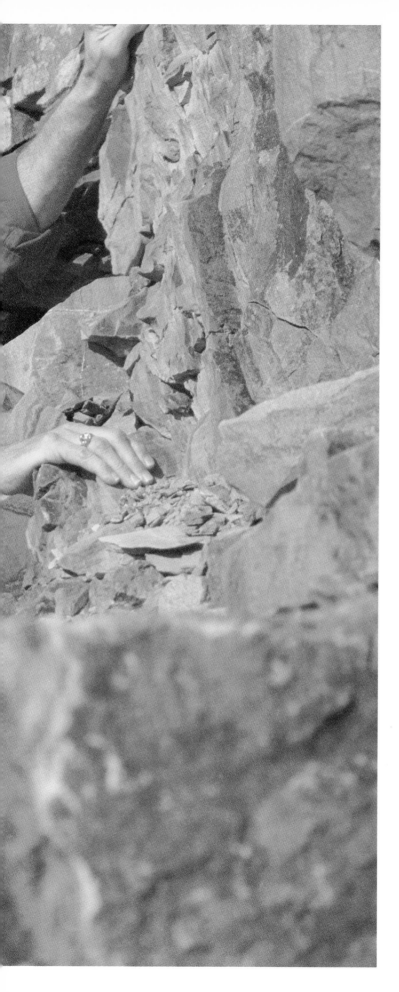

Conquering Chronic Pain

Even though you may not be able to cure the disease, you can control the pain—*today.*

Some pain is so insistent and repetitive it can torture the soul. It may stay for a minute, a week or a month. It may start in one spot, leapfrog from arm to leg to hip or reverberate up and down the length of your spine. It may be sharp or dull. It may be both. It may ache or slice or throb or even burn.

And the minute—the *second*—it disappears, you draw a deep breath all the way to your toes and float through the space it has given you.

But the space is only that. And anxiety, depression and fatigue soon crowd the edges of your moment. You know this is only an interlude. You know that it has a limit. You know that the pain will return.

You also should know that you're not alone. More than one-third of Americans suffer from recurrent pain due to conditions such as blocked arteries, muscle spasms, neurological short-circuits and stressed-out digestive systems.

But such pain can be conquered. It doesn't have to dominate your life so that you spend every moment either waiting for it, suffering from it or gasping in its aftermath. A positive mindset—a refusal to accept a life of pain—along with diet and exercise specifically geared to your body, can frequently prevent even *your* pain. Moreover, a few little tricks that scientists have developed can help you through the attacks you can't prevent and put pain in its proper perspective: It's the symptom, not the disease. Its job is to attract attention to what ails you, not ruin your life.

EASING THE PAIN OF ANGINA

Angina pectoris—a sudden pain, discomfort or tightening in the chest—is one symptom that can be as frightening as it is painful. There is always the fear that the pain isn't just angina at all, but actually the beginning of a heart attack. And,

smoke

Gets in Your Eyes ... And More

Smoky nightclubs may look romantic, but they can lead to heartache. Tobacco smoke contains more than 4,000 compounds, many of which may aggravate angina. And it doesn't matter that you're not the one holding the cigarette. In a study conducted at the Veterans' Administration Medical Center in Long Beach, California, 10 angina patients were twice put in a small room with 3 smokers. During one 2-hour session, the smokers puffed 5 cigarettes each in a well-ventilated room. The next time they smoked the same number of cigarettes over the same time period, but this time the room was unventilated. When researchers compared the smoke sessions, they found that both groups, when exercising, had more rapid onset of angina than usual, with the problem appearing more rapidly among those in the unventilated room.

The lessons for angina sufferers? Avoid smoky rooms, or at least make sure there's an open window.

because in some cases it might be, any pain that lasts longer than 5 to 15 minutes should be investigated by your doctor.

Angina often can be prevented by proper diet, professionally designed exercise programs and learning to handle the everyday aggravations of traffic jams, supermarket lines and people who don't listen when you speak. But before we talk about prevention, let's take a look at just what angina is—and isn't.

Angina occurs when the heart isn't getting enough oxygen. And it demands a lot. With angina the coronary artery is usually blocked with so much sludge that the flow of blood—and its precious oxygen cargo—is reduced to a trickle of less than 40 percent of normal. Or the flow of blood is temporarily blocked by a spasm of the coronary artery.

In either case, blood flow and oxygen availability are usually restored within 5 to 15 minutes. And you can help it along. When angina hits, you should sit down, take a deep breath and relax.

Sound too simple? It's not. Herbert Benson, M.D., a cardiologist and researcher in behavioral medicine at Harvard Medical School and author of *The Relaxation Response* and *Beyond the Relaxation Response*, suggests that an estimated 80 percent of all angina attacks can be relieved as they occur by relaxation combined with what he calls the faith factor. Together these two elements allow you to reduce your heart rate and thus your heart's demand for oxygen.

PICK A WORD, ANY WORD

To develop a relaxation response, Dr. Benson suggests you pick a word or phrase you are comfortable repeating. Any word will do, as long as it invokes your faith (God, Allah, Jesus) or philosophical belief (joy, light, life). Then twice a day—and whenever angina hits—choose a comfortable position, close your eyes, breathe slowly and naturally and relax your muscles, starting with your feet and working up to your head, while focusing on the word or phrase.

Don't worry about extraneous

thoughts or images that keep popping into your consciousness, Dr. Benson advises. They won't affect the meditative process. Just ignore them and continue focusing on your word or phrase.

Stay in this passive state, which is not unlike meditation, between 10 and 20 minutes, advises Dr. Benson. Then sit quietly for another minute, or until you feel like opening your eyes. And don't, Dr. Benson warns, shock your system into awareness by setting the alarm clock to open your eyes. You might just trigger a new attack.

In addition to relaxation, your physician might suggest that you slip a prescription nitroglycerin tablet under your tongue when angina hits. Generally, nitro can be expected to reduce your pain within 1 to 3 minutes by relaxing the walls of veins and arteries within your body. While nitroglycerin is an old standby for treating angina, it can have side effects, including flushing or dizziness. Severe headaches may be an indication of overdose, so be sure to tell your doctor if you get them.

PREVENTION CAN BE EASY

You often can prevent the pain of angina in the first place, however, or keep it from recurring, by lowering the heart's demand for oxygen.

And eating light is a good way to do this. Smaller meals, evenly spaced throughout the day, for example, will detour less oxygen from the heart than the classic three squares a day and a mound of ice cream each night.

The reason is simple. If your meal is heavy in both bulk and calories—roast beef and mashed potatoes with a slice of sweet potato pie would do it—the stomach has to work hard and demands extra oxygen.

If your meal is light—perhaps a cup of tomato soup or a salad—your stomach has little work and its subsequent demands for oxygen are minimal. So the heart can demand—and get—as much oxygen as it needs since the stomach is not pulling away a portion of the body's available oxygen. You can still eat as much as

you need—just eat more frequently throughout the day.

Meals that are lower in fats and calories but higher in eicosapentaenoic acid (EPA)—found in haddock, mackerel, sardines, trout and salmon—may also help the heart get the oxygen it needs.

In a study in Sheffield, England, 92 patients with heart disease were given 10 milliliters of concentrated fish oil—containing less than an ounce of EPA—twice a day. After six months they reported both a decrease in painful angina attacks and an increase in physical capabilities.

KEEP A STEADY BEAT

Almost anything that reduces your heart rate is going to reduce oxygen demand and help prevent angina. Other strategies to keep your heart rate steady include learning not to get bent out of shape over daily problems, consulting your doctor before taking any over-the-counter (OTC) drugs for colds and allergies, preventing anemia, keeping your weight what it should be, cutting out cigarettes and keeping warm. To ease nighttime attacks, raise the head end of your bed 6 to 8 inches. You also can develop—with a professional—an exercise program tailored to your own needs.

Exercise with angina? Indeed. Exercise can help patients manage their angina, according to Victor Froelicher, M.D., chief of cardiology at the Veterans' Administration Medical Center in Long Beach, California. Exercise conditions the heart muscle, says Dr. Froelicher, and forces it to use oxygen more efficiently.

In a Rochester, Minnesota, study, for example, eight angina-prone men between the ages of 45 and 50 participated in a medically supervised exercise program. Over the course of a year, they met with doctors at the local YMCA three times a week for a 45-minute workout. According to their own abilities, they alternately walked and jogged, stretched and either played volleyball or swam. All the men were closely monitored by the doctors.

At the end of a year, each man required less oxygen to do the same

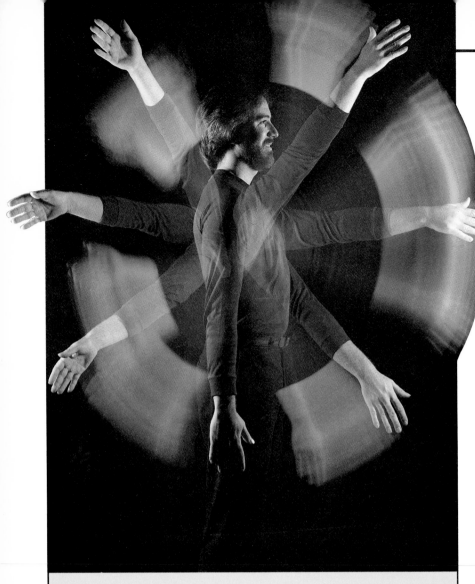

An Exercise to Stop Hand Pain

People who experience the pain of Raynaud's disease, a circulatory problem in which the fingers turn white, then red, might well benefit from an exercise developed by Donald R. McIntyre, M.D., of Vermont.

At the first sign of an attack, swing your arms in a broad circle back and down to one side of your hips, then up in front of your body. Do this at 80 revolutions per minute and gravity and centrifugal force will push blood into your fingers. The increased blood supply will temporarily relieve your pain.

amount of work than when he started the program. And all participants reported a "decrease in angina, an increase in self-esteem, and a more positive attitude toward their work—and their angina."

MIND OVER MATTER

The attitude changes reported in the Rochester study are probably as important as the physical ones.

James L. Levenson, M.D., an assistant professor of psychiatry at the Medical College of Virginia, is convinced that a positive mindset can be as necessary in preventing angina pain as diet and exercise.

"A general observation of surgeons is that patients going into an operation with a negative outlook will probably have a negative outcome," Dr. Levenson says. And this observation also can be applied to angina. The trick is to be realistic about your condition but not let it become a burden.

The executive who conducts business from his hospital bed and has his secretary in for dictation is not being realistic, Dr. Levenson says. Nor is the patient who walks out of a hospital without a much-needed operation.

But the person who accepts the fact that he has often-painful angina pectoris yet refuses to believe it can kill him is probably striking the right balance.

The guiding principle in determining a healthy balance, Dr. Levenson says, is to remember: "Things that you cannot change, put out of your mind."

THE MAGINOT LINE

But some of us are born worriers. We always run worst-case scenarios through our minds at 60 frames a second, then run them back again and find the gore. We think of blood poisoning when we get a blister, gangrene when we get a scratch and funeral processions when we get angina. But don't break out the shovels. If a positive mindset doesn't work for you, diet and exercise probably will. And if *they* don't work, drugs and surgery offer a very real sense of hope.

Both coronary artery bypass surgery, in which blood vessels are borrowed from one part of the body (frequently the leg) to reroute blood around a blocked artery, and "balloon surgery," in which a tiny, deflated balloon catheter is pushed through a clogged artery, inflated slightly and pulled back through the slush to widen the artery, have been successful in preventing the pain of angina.

In a study at London's Hammersmith Hospital, for example, 15 patients who experienced frequent angina underwent bypass surgery. And even though the coronary artery had been at least 70 percent blocked, 14 of them went home with no angina.

Drugs—beta blockers and calcium channel blockers, for example—are also effective in preventing angina (as opposed to treating the attack, like the nitroglycerin discussed earlier). The beta blockers stimulate a complex, biochemical action that refuses to allow your body to get as excited as you do, while the calcium channel blockers dilate blood vessels and moderate heart contractions so the heart doesn't have to work as hard as it normally would to pump blood. Both groups of drugs may cause minor side effects—nausea, dizziness, headache—and occasionally more serious ones such as abnormal heart rhythms, depression, difficulty breathing or impotence.

You can probably work out a drug regimen with your doctor that will minimize these effects. But going for walks, eating lightly, learning to relax and realizing that your glass is half full, not half empty, may be a better deal.

RELIEVING LEG PAIN

Proper diet and exercise are also important in reducing the severity of atherosclerosis, a naturally evolving hardening of the arteries that turns flexible blood vessels into stiff leather.

As we age, arteries grow less elastic. And when combined with the fatty deposits of a fried-egg-and-bacon lifestyle, they are less able to expand and contract as they regulate the flow of blood.

Frequently, this causes a deep ache as blood flow—particularly to the legs—is reduced. But the pain can be relieved by applying heat and resting your legs. An afghan thrown over your calves with a heating pad

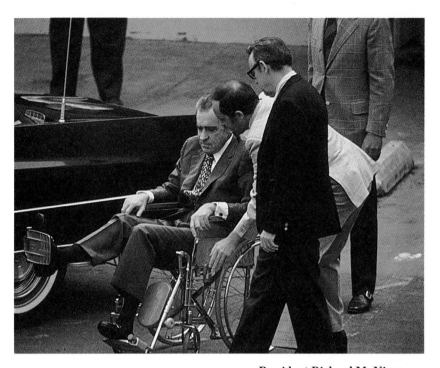

President Richard M. Nixon winces from the pain of phlebitis in 1974. Nixon neglected to tell his doctors when the symptoms first hit, so his medical treatment was delayed.

or a hot compress should be effective, and resting means just that: a temporary pause from labor, not sitting around for half the day.

But if the pain hits your toes—usually a nighttime aggravation—flip your legs over the edge of the bed and wiggle your feet. You may feel a bit foolish, but the increased flow of blood will eliminate your discomfort.

Another condition that affects the legs and can be painful is phlebitis. The condition may affect only superficial veins, causing inflammation, redness and pain, says R. Scott Mitchell, M.D., an assistant professor of cardiovascular surgery at Stanford University Medical Center. It can be relieved by rest, elevation of the leg, local moist heat and aspirin.

A much more serious condition, called thrombophlebitis, involves inflammation of a deep vein and affects the vein's inner lining. Blood clots may form and adhere to the walls of the inflamed vein, or they may even break loose and travel elsewhere. No one knows why they occur. Although the signs of thrombophlebitis may be more subtle than those of phlebitis, you're again saddled with the redness and pain, plus a heaviness and swelling in the affected leg. You may also have chills and a fever.

Doctors do know, says Dr.

Raising Your Bed Can Lower Your Heartburn

You can reduce or eliminate nighttime heartburn by tilting the head end of your bed 6 to 8 inches. You could use blocks or bricks under the legs, but sliding blocks, or worse, sliding beds can be hazardous to your health. Instead, build a slanted box 6 to 8 inches high, just wide enough to rest on the bed frame (see illustration). Make it out of ¾-inch plywood and fasten it to the bottom of the box spring with 1½-inch-long number 8 wood screws. Then plan on a good night's sleep.

Mitchell, that obesity, prolonged sitting, tight clothing such as girdles, varicose veins and tobacco use are risk factors. "Thrombophlebitis is a very serious condition which may be life-threatening," says Dr. Mitchell. If you think you have thrombophlebitis, call your doctor right away because it can cause blood poisoning if left untreated, and a piece of *any* clot can break away and travel to your heart or lungs.

Unfortunately, once you've had thrombophlebitis, you're at higher risk to get it again because the vein never returns to normal, says Dr. Mitchell. But you can reduce the likelihood of recurrence and thus pain: Wear support stockings if you have varicose veins, says Dr. Mitchell, avoid tobacco, maintain your appropriate weight and get regular exercise such as walking.

HOW DO *YOU* SPELL RELIEF?

Unfortunately, it's not as easy to prevent the recurrence of heartburn. This chronically painful problem is frequently described by the one-third of all Americans who suffer from it as "that burning sensation." And well it deserves such an incendiary description. Physicians who use special tools called endoscopes to look right at the inflamed esophagus say that the inflammation of this hoselike structure is painfully clear. But the "burn" is caused by irritation from the repeated backwash of food, acid and enzymes from your stomach into the esophagus, not by flames.

Occasionally the backwash is triggered by a hiatal hernia, a condition in which the top of the stomach pokes through an opening in the diaphragm. When the stomach tries to squish itself through the hole, it can force open the lower esophageal sphincter (LES)—a valvelike band of muscle that forms the opening between esophagus and stomach. And that encourages the stomach's contents to rise toward the throat, leaving you in pain.

If the LES is weak due to the strain of pregnancy or obesity or other causes, it can also relax at the wrong moment and allow the stomach's contents to flow back up

the esophagus. And it's particularly prone to do so when you're bending over, slumping in a chair, lying down or in any way not vertically lined up with the gravitational pull of the planet.

"Most people take an Alka-Seltzer and lie down" when heartburn hits, says Barbara Bachman, M.D., a former Mayo Clinic researcher who is now at the University of South Florida. "What they *should* do," she emphasizes, "is take a liquid antacid and sit *up*."

Sitting up will reduce pressure against the LES, explains Dr. Bachman, and help keep it from opening at the wrong moment. Antacids will soothe the stomach and actually tighten the sphincter. Moreover, if taken in liquid form, says Dr. Bachman, antacids can coat the esophagus and provide topical relief as well.

SAVE A BUCK

But which antacid is best?

Most antacids are fast, effective and relatively safe for an occasional dose after holiday dinners. But they are not for regular, daily consumption. For example, don't do what the associate dean of a college in Philadelphia used to do. He kept a pack of cigarettes, a roll of antacid tablets and a cup of coffee lined up on his desk, next to the blotter. Throughout the day, he'd take a sip of coffee and pop an antacid, smoke a cigarette and pop an antacid, have an argument with the dean and pop an antacid. By the end of his 14-hour day, his eyes were popping out of his head. This is self-abuse, because almost all antacids have side effects when overdosed. Calcium carbonate, a good acid neutralizer, can cause constipation when used more than six times a week. And if you have kidney disease, both calcium carbonate and magnesium hydroxide can cause serious complications. But, if used according to directions, antacids are all right—and can be very helpful.

One antacid, however, doesn't work well alone and can cause problems. Aluminum hydroxide, the least effective of the antacids, can—even in small doses—cause constipation and bone demineralization. Fortu-

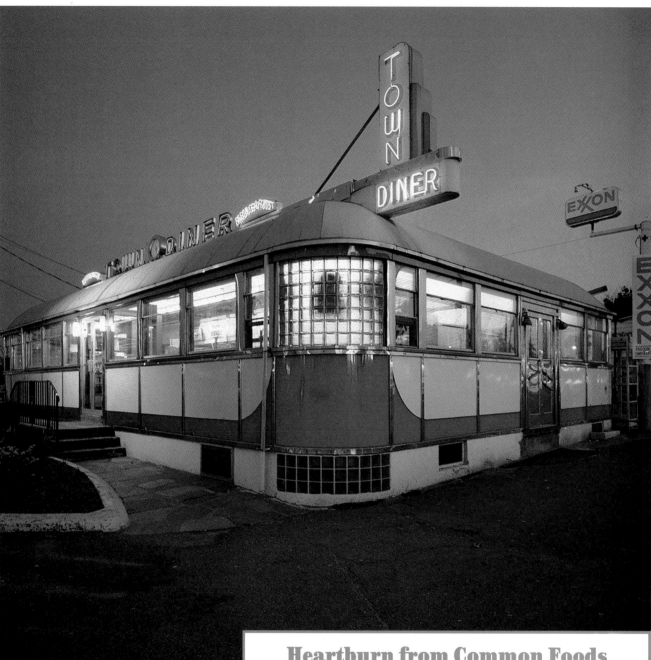

Heartburn from Common Foods

"Greasy spoons" deserve a break. They aren't to blame for your heartburn—you are. Because it's *what* you eat, not *where* you eat it that causes pain. Some foods that may trigger heartburn include carbonated beverages, pastry, cake icing, spearmint, peppermint, citrus juices, coffee, fatty or spicy foods, alcohol and chocolate. But not everyone has a problem with each of these foods. Experiment. Find your heartburn trigger—and then avoid pulling it.

nately, it is usually combined with magnesium hydroxide or sodium carbonate to reduce the chance of constipation. Bone demineralization, however, remains a problem.

PREVENTING THE PAIN

So when heartburn hits, you figure out which antacid is best for *you* and go for it, right?

Well, maybe. But maybe not. There are a few alternatives that may act like antacids but without those occasionally irritating side effects. Some people, for example, report

that algin, an extract of the seaweed kelp, reduces heartburn. Others say that drinking water or eating garlic and parsley tablets, papaya tablets, parsley, alfalfa sprouts or celery helps *them*. There's no scientific proof for any of these treatments. But as long as you don't throw these suggestions into some kind of weird Bloody Mary or on top of a pizza, they probably won't hurt, and they just might work.

But there's not much point in taking antacids or celery or both to relieve heartburn and tighten the LES if you're going to turn right around and eat things that will just loosen the sphincter again.

Fatty foods, caffeinated beverages, "decaffeinated" beverages (which still, the commercials forget to tell you, have some caffeine), chocolate, citrus fruits, tobacco smoke and large meals are all prime LES looseners, says Dr. Bachman. And so are vitamin C supplements. If you have heartburn but still want to take vitamin C supplements, says Dr. Bachman, take a multivitamin that contains C rather than taking plain ascorbic acid. The multivitamin combination doesn't give the same instant heartburn as a direct shot of C to the esophagus.

Other drugs, including antihistamines, can cause heartburn. So if yours persists, ask your doctor if it might be caused by any drugs you are taking.

Moreover, if you know your heartburn is triggered by a hiatal hernia, wear loose clothes and eat lots of fiber so you won't have to strain when you defecate. And don't eat less than 2 hours before going to bed.

DROWN YOUR ULCER PAIN

People with ulcers also might want to avoid eating before bed, because that soothing little snack right before taps will cause your stomach to secrete extra acid. The result is a burning pain around 1:00 or 2:00 A.M. as your stomach or upper intestine begins eating away at itself.

Years ago, doctors would have advised you to reach for a glass of

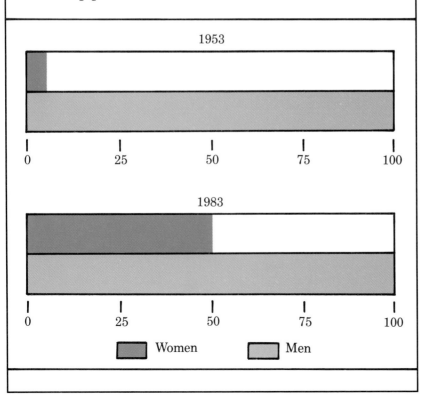

Women Gain (a Painful) Equality

You've come a long way, baby—but maybe you should check your direction. A study of 82 ulcer patients at the University of Auckland, New Zealand, revealed that the ratio of male to female stomach ulcers is now 2 to 1, while 30 years ago it was 20 to 1. No one knows exactly why the tenfold increase has occurred, but a significant factor may be cigarettes, which inhibit the body's ability to neutralize stomach acid. Since more women smoke, the theory goes, more women may develop painful ulcers.

1953

| 0 | 25 | 50 | 75 | 100 |

1983

| 0 | 25 | 50 | 75 | 100 |

☐ Women ☐ Men

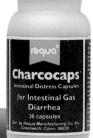

milk to ease the pain. But today they know that the high protein content of milk actually exacerbates acid secretion, resulting in worse pain than you started with.

Instead of milk, most doctors suggest you take liquid antacids. And not just when the pain hits. Aside from taking drugs like cimetidine (Tagamet), which reduces acid secretion and is prescribed to help heal and prevent recurrences of duodenal ulcers, the most effective way to relieve ulcer pain immediately is to take antacids. One gastroenterologist (a digestion specialist) recommends you drown your ulcer in 2 tablespoons of an antacid like Mylanta II 1 hour after meals, again 2 hours later and also at bedtime. Continue the regimen for six weeks. Because of the possible side effects mentioned previously, that's the maximum therapy, although a lower dose may work.

If you have a little rumbling once in a while, take a single shot of antacid, says the gastroenterologist. But if ulcer pain hits three times a week or more, it's time for a full-fledged response, because your ulcer is worsening. Left untreated it can continue eating away at your stomach or intestinal lining until it bores a hole through the tissue and penetrates neighboring blood vessels, organs or glands.

The pain at this point is exquisite. It may slice through the upper stomach or abdominal area, but it promptly spreads over the entire abdomen. Any movement is painful. Fever, rapid heartbeat and shock may ensue and immediate medical attention is necessary. Surgery, with a

mortality rate up to 10 percent, is required when the stomach is perforated.

Clearly, treating an ulcer and minimizing the chances it will recur are important—particulary since most ulcers *do* return. But aside from avoiding milk, you can even the odds by also avoiding other ulcer irritants such as baking soda, aspirin (even buffered), and any foods that past experience says will upset your stomach. No special diet is necessary and (contrary to popular opinion) spicy foods aren't more likely to cause ulcer pain than any other food.

And don't smoke. Although no one really knows what causes ulcers, smoking is the most powerful risk factor.

A study of 370 recently healed patients, for example, revealed that ulcers recurred more often in those who smoked, regardless of whether they received medication or placebos (fake pills). And a second study demonstrated that high-dose antacids healed 67 percent of duodenal ulcers in nonsmokers, but only 39 percent of the ulcers in smokers. So not only can smoking influence ulcer recurrence, it also may affect the ability of antacids to aid in healing.

Smoking also inhibits the effectiveness of cimetidine. In one study, 34 percent of those ulcer patients who smoked and took cimetidine reported painful ulcer recurrence. Yet only 18 percent of those who took cimetidine and *didn't* smoke reported further pain. Whether or not someone smokes, concluded the researchers, is more likely to determine ulcer recurrence than whether or not they take an ulcer drug like cimetidine.

Better Than Gas

Flatulence is a humorous subject only on stages and playgrounds. At home and at work, or out with friends, it's a pain. But Raymond G. Hall, Jr., Ph.D., a researcher at Loma Linda University in California, claims that activated charcoal—the kind found at your drugstore, not in your barbecue pit—may offer some relief.

Dr. Hall fed 30 volunteers gas-producing meals (including foods such as those shown above), then divided them into 2 groups. One group was given activated charcoal, the other group a placebo. The charcoal group had significantly less gas. If you decide to give it a try, remember that it's not for extended, daily use.

Alternatives to Hemorrhoid Surgery

Hemorrhoid surgery has come a long way since the kings of France used unskilled proctologists to hack off their hemorrhoids without anesthesia. But it still requires a painful, 6-week recovery period. Yet hemorrhoid surgery is necessary only when pain and bleeding persist and hemorrhoids drop down through the anus and stay there, says David A. Lieberman, M.D., a gastroenterologist at Oregon Health Sciences University. Otherwise, says Dr. Lieberman, the treatment of choice is rubber band ligation, an outpatient procedure in which a band is slipped on a small portion of the hemorrhoid, causing it to drop off (usually painlessly) a week or so later. Other alternatives you can ask your doctor about include anal dilation, hemorrhoidal injections, freezing or infrared coagulation.

STRESS CAUSES BOWEL PAIN

One thing that has never really been *proven* to cause ulcer recurrence, however, is stress—although it does play an important part in another type of digestive pain, irritable bowel syndrome (IBS). With IBS, hypersensitive cells lining the intestine produce a lot of pain during normal intestinal contractions.

Unfortunately, IBS pain frequently mimics the pain of an ulcer. It is not unusual for people to think they have ulcers when they really have IBS or to think they have IBS when they really have ulcers. And since IBS can be a response to stress, that *may* explain why so many people who think they have ulcers—when they don't—think that their ulcers are triggered by stress—when they aren't. It's also why people need to see their doctor for a proper diagnosis.

But what actually causes IBS pain is muscle spasm and trapped gas. Pinch a tube of toothpaste at one end, then squeeze it at both ends. The middle bulges out, right? Now think of that tube of toothpaste as your intestinal tract. The squeezing represents muscle spasms, which cause pain, and the area that bulges out is trapped gas, which also causes pain.

Now to relieve the pain, you have to relax the muscle spasms and free the trapped gas. And the way to do that, one doctor suggests, is to get up and move around, take a tablet of simethicone (or an antacid with that ingredient), which cuts down on the gas, then excuse yourself from company, go to the bathroom, and try to push the rest of the gas out of your body. Above all, he says, "Don't panic. The pain always gets better."

There is one technique, however, that may speed things along and prevent recurrence: hypnosis (see chapter 9). Researchers at University Hospital of South Manchester in England studied 26 women and 4 men with severe IBS, all of whom experienced abdominal pain, gas, diarrhea, constipation, or alternating diarrhea and constipation. And even though they had been under treatment for at least a year, nothing had relieved their pain.

The researchers divided the study participants into two groups. One group received a placebo and seven ½-hour sessions of psychotherapy aimed at reducing stress. The second group received seven ½-hour sessions of hypnotherapy that helped participants to relax the smooth muscle tissue of the intestine. They also received a cassette tape that they could use to hypnotize themselves at home on a daily basis.

At the end of the three-month treatment period, the hypnosis group had either no pain or gas or very little, and a significant improvement in bowel habits. The psychotherapy group reported a small but significant lessening in pain and gas, and no change in the frequency of diarrhea or constipation or both.

No one knows why hypnosis works, the researchers concluded; they just know that it does. But they suspect that rather than creating a psychological effect, it may work directly on the intestine to relax muscle spasms. IBS is not, in other words, all in your head. It really is in your gut—just like you've been telling people all along. That may mean that you can hypnotize your gut into submission and merrily trip through the rest of your life. But there are doctors who point out that IBS is occasionally a symptom of food allergy or even an indication of severe dietary fiber depletion. A food exclusion test under your doctor's supervision will reveal the former and a diet rich in whole grains, veggies and fruits will stop the latter.

HEMORRHOIDS: THE FIBER FACTOR

Fiber also may stop hemorrhoid pain. Hemorrhoids, which are swollen veins that may or may not protrude from the anus, are painful only when they are protruding, swollen and inflamed. And they can be absolutely excruciating when they are roughed-up during a hard bowel movement.

In fact, "many people shy away from having a bowel movement" because of the pain, says Leon Banov, Jr., M.D., a Charlestown, South Carolina, proctologist and former adviser to the U.S. Food and

Drug Administration. But they shouldn't. Hemorrhoid pain is easily relieved, says Dr. Banov, by analgesics such as aspirin or Tylenol, a stool softener such as Surfak, the use of wet pads of absorbent cotton instead of dry toilet paper, bed rest and an occasional enema.

Note, emphasizes Dr. Banov, the use of the word *occasional* with the word *enema*. Some people feel they need to have at least one bowel movement every day, but that's not true. Each person has his own schedule. And trying to force your body to a schedule not of its inclination can, in Dr. Banov's words, have "explosive" results. Particularly if you also use laxatives, which are thought by some doctors to actually *aggravate* hemorrhoid problems by causing too many bowel movements.

An easier way to promote softer and less painful bowel movements, says David A. Lieberman, M.D., a gastroenterologist and assistant professor of medicine at Oregon Health Sciences University, is to add a few tablespoons of bran to your diet each day. In one or two days, as the bowel movements soften and become easier, says Dr. Lieberman, the pain may lessen.

To ensure getting enough fiber, substitute whole grain breads and cereals for refined ones and take 1 tablespoon of a bulking agent such as Metamucil three times a day. And, to be perfectly blunt, says Dr. Lieberman, "Take it to the point that the stool is soft and mushy." The stools of rural Africans who eat large amounts of seeds, nuts, whole grains and other types of fiber are the consistency of oatmeal, Dr. Lieberman points out. And the Africans rarely have hemorrhoids.

NO STRAIN, NO PAIN

Softer stools should eliminate the need for straining during bowel movements. And straining in combination with hard stools can actually cause an anal fissure—a small tear in the anal canal that is exquisitely painful. Small fissures will eventually heal themselves, says Dr. Lieberman. But until they do, periodically sitting on a child-sized inner tube in a tub of warm water may relieve the pain—

just as it does for hemorrhoids.

An over-the-counter hemorrhoidal ointment with an anesthetic such as benzocaine (Lanacaine, Medicone, Nupercainal) or pramoxine hydrochloride (Tronolane, Anusol) may also help, adds Dr. Banov. But OTC ointments are not effective in all cases of anorectal disorders. One problem is that people don't apply them correctly, Dr. Banov explains. You have to remember that an anal fissure is not as prominently located as a hemorrhoid. So just smearing some ointment over the area is useless. To apply an emollient correctly, in cases of a fissure, says Dr. Banov, you need to spread the buttocks apart with one hand so that the fissure is more likely to be exposed, then apply the ointment directly to the area with the other hand.

Read the ointment's label for information on length of treatment, advises Dr. Banov, and don't exceed the manufacturer's recommendation. Otherwise, you might become sensitive to the ointment and end up with more pain than when you started.

Dr. Lieberman agrees. There have been no carefully controlled studies that proved whether or not OTC preparations work for regular hemorrhoids. Hydrocortisone, a drug that reduces swelling and inflammation, is contained in some of the preparations. But it's in minute amounts, and its role is unproven, says Dr. Lieberman. The main job of OTC preparations, he adds, is to coat and protect the anal area, which is why they contain so many emollients.

You might also avoid sitting on the toilet for prolonged periods, since that puts pressure on your hemorrhoids, suggests Dr. Banov. And avoid using dry toilet paper and excessive rubbing.

Dry toilet paper just spreads fecal matter and rubbing irritates the whole area. "If you have mud on your forehead," Dr. Banov points out, "you wouldn't rub *it* in." So whether you have an anal fissure or just plain hemorrhoids, cleanse after bowel movements by folding and wetting the toilet paper or wetting absorbent cotton and blotting the area. Don't rub. Water cleans better than dry paper. Or use moist medicated pads from the drugstore.

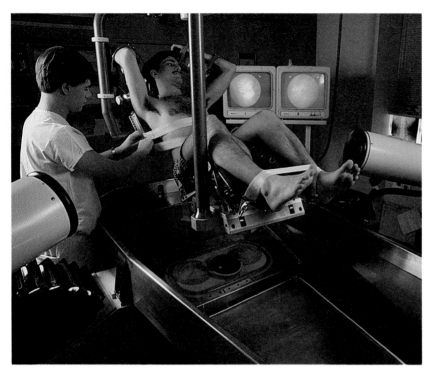

Z-z-z-z-z-z-zap! This somewhat torturous-looking device was created by Dr. Christian Chaussey with a team of associates from the University of Munich, and it may be a godsend for those who form painful kidney stones. With high-voltage electrical sparks that create shock waves in a tank of water, the machine, called a lithotripter, smashes kidney stones into small fragments. These are then flushed out of the body along with urine—a far cry from the typical pain-wracked expulsion. With the patient under anesthesia, the lithotripter procedure takes about 30 to 45 minutes and a report—like the crack of a gunshot—zaps across the room with each spark. The sparks are timed to miss coinciding with your heartbeat, so the shock won't cause an abnormal beat. All this excitement may soon be a thing of the past, however, because a new type of lithotripter, which uses lasers rather than electric sparks, is being developed to avoid the possibility of such a shock.

And remember, advises Dr. Lieberman, pain is a signal that something is wrong. If the fiber diet, warm soak and OTC emollient don't help things along, give your doctor a call. Significant pain may mean a significant problem. Get it checked.

THE PIERCING PAIN OF GALLSTONES

Gallstones, which are usually multifaceted clumps of excess cholesterol found in the gallbladder, can form silently over a lifetime.

Silently, that is, until a shaft of pain pierces the upper right side of your abdomen—or between your shoulder blades—as a stone drops into the bile duct leading from gallbladder to intestine. Imagine trying to force a chip of stone through a thin rubber tube and you've got the general idea. And the only way to stop the pain is to move the stone.

There isn't a lot you can do on your own. Some doctors suggest that you go to bed, take a prescribed painkiller, sip water, avoid food and pray that the stone either falls back into the gallbladder or makes it to the intestine.

But if the pain persists for more

than 3 hours, chances are that it's stuck. And when it's stuck, explains Gerald Salen, M.D., a researcher at the East Orange Veterans' Medical Center in New Jersey, surgical removal of the stone—and usually your gallbladder with it—is the only way to stop the pain.

If the stone does drop back into the gallbladder, however, you may get a second chance. Mayo Clinic researchers are studying methyl test-butyl ether (MTBE) as a possible stone-dissolving agent, while the drug chenodiol (Chenix) has already been proven to dissolve a small portion of the softer, less crystalline gallstones. And in a study of 200 people, Dr. Salen found that urso-deoxycholic acid (a component of bear bile) dissolved the stones in 50 percent of his patients. Often the pain associated with gallstones was relieved in about one week. However, if the pain was caused by inflammation of the gallbladder, then surgery was the only effective treatment.

No one is thrilled to have to choose between only surgery and drugs, but either one is a better choice than ignoring the gallstone, because leaving gallstones untreated can be dangerous as well as painful. Left in the bile duct, a stone can cause inflammation and infection. The gallbladder will swell, pain will increase, your temperature will rise, and nausea and vomiting may follow. And if you *still* don't seek treatment, the gallbladder itself may burst—setting off one firecracker of an infection. At that point the only decision you have to make is which surgeon should do the cutting.

There are ways, however, to keep from getting to that point. Reducing the cholesterol content of your bloodstream through a low-fat diet and exercise has been a standard approach for years. And despite a study at Georgetown University that indicated that—like the ulcer diet of yore—low-fat diets may not be as effective as scientists had hoped in treating gallstones that have not caused pain, these diets probably continue to be recommended. One major reason for this is that gallstone "attacks" frequently occur after a fatty meal. Another is that it is known that fat people, who frequently consume a

Margarita Coldwell
New York, N.Y.
Carpal Tunnel Syndrome

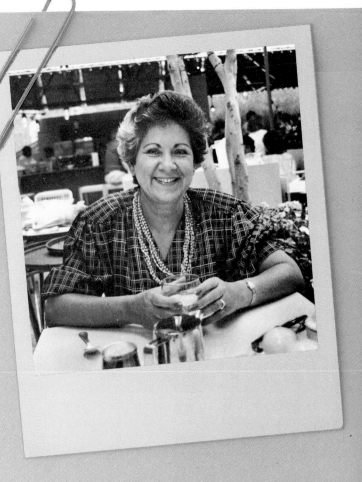

Seated beneath a pink umbrella at the Festival Cafe in Manhattan, a tanned and smiling Margarita Coldwell does not look like someone who spent 6 nearly sleepless months unable to move her hand without pain. But as a victim of carpal tunnel syndrome (CTS), a disease in which the nerve passing through the wrist is—for a variety of reasons—pinched by surrounding tissues, Margarita is fortunate to be pain free today. Many CTS victims are not.

"I started by having a little pin sensation biting the tips of my fingers," explains Margarita, whose soft accent reflects her South American heritage. "Then I noticed that I could not make a fist." She clenches a hand in front of her. "If I held some coins in my hand," she says as she opens her fingers, "they'd slip out because I couldn't close it."

Margarita shrugs. "I went to see several doctors, including one in Costa Rica. Three of them told me that I had to have an operation. But people kept on telling me, 'Oh, Margarita, don't have the operation done, some people get worse, some people—instead of a hand they get sort of a claw—things like that." Margarita shakes her head. "I was scared to death."

Finally, she went to see Richard Eaton, M.D., director of hand surgery at St. Luke's-Roosevelt Hospital in New York. Dr. Eaton also recommended surgery and, convinced at last, Margarita was on her way to the operating room.

On an outpatient basis, and with a local anesthetic, the operation took about 2 hours from the initial incision to the last smear of plaster on her cast. It was not painful, Margarita claims, and after the anesthetic wore off she was given pain medication to take home. She didn't need much, she says, and within a week she was back at Aerolineas Argentinas, the Argentine airline where she has worked for 28 years.

"Of course," Margarita admits, "I could not do anything with my hands because the cast came all the way from the knuckles to above the elbow." But 2 weeks later the cast, the pain and the fear of deformity were gone. Margarita's hand was well.

Now, 2 years after the whole traumatic experience, Margarita sits at the Festival Cafe, one brightly manicured hand curled around a water glass, the other playing with the strings of turquoise around her neck. Her hands look strong and flexible. You have to know just where to look in order to find the scars. Has she had any pain since the operation?

"No," she says simply. "None at all."

high-fat diet, are twice as likely to form gallstones as those who maintain their appropriate weight.

But doctors may also begin recommending diets that are high in fiber and low in refined sugars. Researchers in Italy who studied gallstone formation in 320 people over a five-year period concluded that study participants who had gallstones ate more refined sugars and less vegetables and fruit than those without them. And, half a world away, a researcher at the University of Alberta found that people who regularly ate bran cereal literally spring-cleaned their gallbladders of cholesterol.

When you eat, however, may be just as important as *what* you eat. In another study, this one in France, physicians found that many of a group of 47 women with gallstones either skipped breakfast or waited an abnormally long time between dinner and their next meal. That extended period between meals—which the body treats as a minifast—apparently causes the gallbladder to lose the inclination to store cholesterol-absorbing bile. The result is a supersaturated bile in which excess cholesterol is more likely to settle out into soft lumps, clump together and solidify into gallstones. Clearly, skipping meals is *not* the way to avoid the pain of gallstones.

KIDNEY STONES ARE WORSE

But as painful as gallstones may be, kidney stones are worse. "Kidney stones are God's way of letting men know what birth is like," says Richard Berger, M.D., chief urologist at the University of Washington's Harborview Hospital.

And he's not joking. Kidney stone pain, which comes when a stone pushes its way out of the kidney and along a tube leading to the bladder, is excruciating. Aspirin, indomethacin (Indocin) or ibuprofen (Motrin) may reduce the amount of pain, says Dr. Berger, and pressing on your back near the lumbar vertebra (the same spot described in the caption on page 71) has been known to help—at least while you're pressing.

But the pain will not go away completely until you get rid of the stone—either by passing it in your urine, having it removed by one of several surgical or pseudosurgical procedures or having it shattered by electrically generated shock waves (see the photo on page 64). Typically, the only stones that can be dissolved by medication are stones formed from uric acid or an infection, or cystine stones, in which case drugs,

---

Hip Pocket Sciatica

Even prosperity can give you a pain in the behind! A traveling businessman who suffered "sciatica" for over a year could find no relief. Some specialists blamed a ruptured disk for the shooting pains running down the back of his left leg, but Elmar G. Lutz, M.D., of Passaic, New Jersey, discovered the true "seat" of the problem—the overstuffed wallet the patient carried in his back pocket. "Walletectomy resulted in fairly immediate and complete relief," quipped Dr. Lutz.

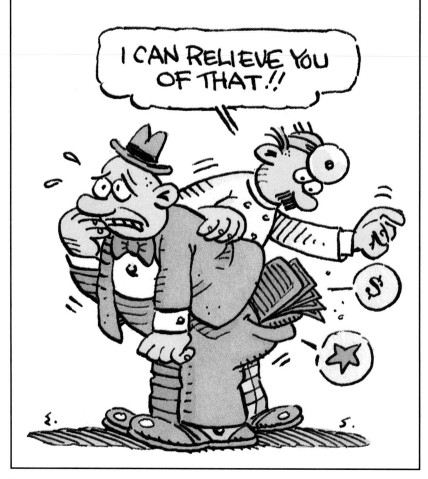

including antibiotics, can solve the problem.

Unfortunately, most stones are formed from calcium oxalate or calcium phosphate. And if you want to prevent their recurrence—they recur in two-thirds of those who get them to begin with—drink lots of water (8 to 12 glasses a day), avoid salt and have any stones you have passed analyzed at a hospital laboratory so that you can adjust your diet accordingly.

If the stones are made of calcium oxalate, for example, you may want to reduce your intake of oxalate-rich foods: grapefruit, cocoa, spinach and rhubarb. Some researchers also suggest that vitamin B_6 (pyridoxine) may reduce the amount of oxalic acid excreted in your urine, while others indicate that magnesium supplements can have a similar effect. (Ask your doctor if you should take these supplements.)

In addition to any dietary changes, you may also consider increasing the amount you exercise. There is some evidence that indicates that exercise may prevent calcium oxalate crystals from remaining in the kidney, where they can crystallize into painful stones.

Activity levels also affect the formation of calcium phosphate stones, says Dr. Berger. If you're an athlete who is laid up for a while with an injury, the lack of exercise can actually cause large amounts of calcium to leach out of your bones and accumulate in your urine. And more calcium in the urine means more chance that stones will form.

In this situation, or if you're someone who regularly forms calcium stones, drink water until your urine becomes clear, says Dr. Berger. And lower the amount of calcium in your diet by limiting dairy products to no more than two servings a day. (Do not avoid dairy products altogether, however. This can lead to nutritional deficiencies.)

SCIATICA RELIEF: FIND THE CAUSE

Unfortunately, there's nothing you can eliminate from your diet to make the sciatic nerve stop quivering once it's been zapped. From its roots deep

Exercise Sciatica Away

One of the best ways to build up abdominal muscles and thus both prevent and treat the crippling spasms that frequently cause sciatica is to make love—regularly, leisurely and tenderly, says Lawrence W. Friedmann, M.D., in his book *Freedom from Backaches.* But if there's no bed—or partner—handy when sciatica hits, try one of these exercises.

Hip Rotation

Tilt your pelvis toward the wall in front of you. Rotate it around smoothly to the right, back, left and front. Reverse direction. Repeat several times. Breathe deeply.

Spinal Twist

Sit straight on a chair or on the floor. Turn your head and upper body to the left. Grasp your left thigh with your right hand. Pull on your thigh to give your torso a good twist. Rest your left arm on the floor or chair back for support. Reverse and repeat the exercise, exhaling as you twist to each side.

Lower Back Twist

Lie on your back with your knees bent, feet flat and hands on the floor. Exhale as you drop your knees to the left and turn your head to the right. Inhale as you bring your knees back upright. Exhale as you let your knees roll to the right, moving your head left. Repeat several times.

inside the spine and pelvis, across the buttocks, down the back of your thigh, knee and calf, right down to the foot—it's going to tingle and ache and burn.

Most sciatic pain can be alleviated by bed rest (on a firm but not rigid mattress), regular exercise (see "Exercise Sciatica Away" on page 67), massage (especially if some of the pain is due to a muscle spasm), analgesics (aspirin, ibuprofen), hot baths (20 to 30 minutes), spinal manipulation (by an osteopath or physiatrist) and acupressure—for example, locate one point on your hip and another on your calf, then push hard for 30 seconds. (You'll know you've got the right points if the pain lessens.) Steroid and local anesthetic injections are helpful somewhere between 60 and 73 percent of the time. If these fail, surgery may be indicated.

Although the main cause of sciatica is a herniated disk, it also can be attributed to causes that range from muscle spasms that pinch the nerve to tumors to fat wallets to slanted car seats to sitting with your knees straight instead of bent. The key is to keep looking for the cause until you find it, because that's when you'll get rid of your pain.

THE GUESSWORK OF TIC DOULOUREUX

The cause of pain along another of the body's nerve paths, the trigeminal nerve, is more likely to remain a mystery. In fact, so little is actually understood about this nerve—which carries tiny networks of sensation from forehead to chin along both sides of the face—that at least one doctor flatly says that almost all treatment of tic douloureux ("painful twitch"), the syndrome in which a burning pain zaps down the victim's face without warning, is experimental.

But experimental or not, there is promising research being done. There are some indications that the anticonvulsive drug Tegretol can, in some cases, relieve the pain, says Christopher F. Terrence, M.D., a neurologist at the Pittsburgh Veterans' Medical Center. And an experimental use of an old drug, Baclofen, on

which he and his colleague Gerhard Fromm, M.D., are working, may be even better.

Although studies are based on only a handful of people, it seems that Baclofen may be able to help at least 60 percent of those who suffer from tic. One 70-year-old woman, for example, hadn't eaten in ten days because swallowing triggered her pain. She lost 10 to 15 pounds before she was finally referred to Dr. Terrence and Dr. Fromm. They put her on the Baclofen and her pain disappeared. At last report she was merrily gaining back her lost weight.

But when tic douloureux drug therapies fail—or the side effects such as nausea, dizziness, fatigue and bone marrow problems can't be handled—it's time to consult a surgeon. There are a number of surgical techniques that can relieve tic douloureux pain, says Russel H. Patterson, Jr., M.D., a professor of surgery and neurosurgery at Cornell Medical Center. Most of these involve trading off a degree of facial sensation for a degree of pain relief. The most effective and least destructive technique, he says, is microsurgical decompression, an operation in which a sponge is inserted between the trigeminal nerve and any neighboring vein or artery that may be periodically putting pressure on the nerve. If it sounds as though no one is really sure whether or not nerve compression causes tic, that's because they aren't. But they do know that the procedure relieves pain in 78 to 90 percent of the patients who undergo it. The recurrence rate is perhaps 10 percent of the cases and some hearing loss may result. Microsurgical decompression *is* major surgery, emphasizes Dr. Patterson, and it is only for those in good health.

But tic douloureux victims who are not in the best health have other options. In studies, transcutaneous electrical nerve stimulation (TENS), discussed in chapter 10, and radiofrequency coagulation, a procedure that actually involves burning the trigeminal nerve, seemed to be helpful in about half the patients on whom they were performed. And in another study, surgical injections of glycerol relieved pain in 67 percent of tic douloureux victims. Recurrent pain is not unusual with any of these procedures, however.

Of course, sometimes even a day free of pain is worth the risk. Especially with a pain so bad that it is triggered by washing your face.

DON'T SUFFER WITH SHINGLES

People with severe cases of shingles aren't usually as disabled by their pain as people with tic douloureux, but "some are out of their minds by the time they come to me," says S. Harvey Sklar, M.D., of the agony that shingles can bring.

The virus lives hidden away in your body after a childhood bout with chicken pox (shingles and chicken pox are both members of the herpes family), explains Dr. Sklar, who is the senior attending physician in pediatrics at Englewood Hospital in New Jersey and a consultant to the hospital's shingles clinic.

Then when something as innocuous as a cold or physical trauma or just getting a day older activates the virus, it starts traveling along the nerve in which it's been hiding. That causes the pain. The skin rash, which is characterized by clear blisters that eventually pop, ooze and disappear, develops along the nerve fiber's surface path—literally marking the virus's progress within your body.

Traditional treatment of shingles —primarily nerve blocks, biofeedback, antidepressants, TENS, hypnosis, sedatives and narcotics—has been aimed at helping the shingles victim bear the pain until the body's natural defenses build up enough strength to attack the virus and send it back into hiding. But for at least 60 percent of shingles victims between the ages of 60 and 69, says Dr. Sklar, sustained nerve cell damage may lead to chronic pain. The pain can stay at least a month, or six months, or a year, or even forever.

Unfortunately, this kind of chronic pain, what doctors call postherpetic neuralgia, has been impossible to prevent or treat. People have just had to live with it. But in a study recently completed by Dr. Sklar and his associates, 15 of 17 patients who were given adenosine monophosphate (AMP), a by-product of metabolism, were free of pain within 14 days. At the same time, only 6 of 15 patients receiving placebos were pain free. "After four weeks all patients who had not recovered from pain started receiving AMP treatment," according to Dr. Sklar. Then their pain disappeared within three weeks. And in a two-year follow-up, not one patient successfully treated with AMP had a single moment of pain.

But the key to AMP's success, warns Dr. Sklar, is early treatment. Beyond the fifth month of shingles, nerve cells are so damaged that even AMP is ineffective. And the only relief from pain then is the sometimes fogged-out never-never land of narcotics. As one doctor says, "Sometimes all you can do is give them narcotics and sympathy."

THE COLD FACTS
ABOUT CRAMPS

Sympathy is one thing you don't get when you've got painful cramps. Instead, women get handed a heating pad and a box full of Kotex the day they turn 12, plus an earful of myths ranging from "Cramps are the revenge of an unfilled womb" to "Tampons will ruin your virginity" to "Don't go swimming—it will stop your period" to "Running will make your uterus fall out."

Sound wild? It's no wilder than a study that reports that 39 percent of the men and 31 percent of the women surveyed feel that a woman's thinking is impaired during her period. Nor is it wilder than the fact that gynecology has become an elective subject in some medical schools. And it may tend to explain why research into cramps has historically been somewhat less than helpful.

But solutions are being discovered—sometimes in unusual ways. One group of Canadian women, for example, noticed that those in the group who worked in slaughterhouses seemed to get menstrual cramps more often and more severely than women in their community who worked at home.

But why? To find out, the women turned to Donna Mergler, Ph.D., a member of the Research Group in Occupational Health at the University of Quebec in Montreal.

Dr. Mergler and an associate

studied 213 women who worked at the slaughterhouses and 105 women who worked at home. They found that cramps were so severe in women who worked in the slaughterhouses that almost one-quarter of them were forced to go home during their periods. And an examination of various factors in their workplaces caused Dr. Mergler to zero in on the temperature.

A comparison of temperature, work station and pain revealed that 14 percent of the women at "warm" work stations, 20 percent of those at "cold" stations and 33 percent of those at "very cold" stations "took sick leave during their last menstrual period." It seems that as the temperature dropped, everyone's cramps increased significantly. Normally, as Dr. Mergler pointed out in her study, only 10 percent of any particular group of women will be incapacitated by menstrual cramps, whether they're school girls or nurses or welders. Clearly, cold seems to increase the pain of cramps.

But—besides pulling on a long sweater, some wool trousers and a pair of knitted snow-bunny boots— what can you do when cramps start squeezing your guts?

Exercise, making love, vitamin E and calcium are all believed by some people to help cramps. But many doctors also suggest nonsteroidal anti-inflammatory drugs such as ibuprofen (Motrin) or naproxen (Anaprox). And that advice reflects the latest theory as to why women get cramps: They produce excess amounts of prostaglandin (a hormonelike substance made from essential fatty acids) during their periods. The prostaglandin is believed to stimulate excessive uterine contractions which, in turn, cause the pain.

No one knows whether or not this theory is more accurate than any other. What scientists do know, however, is that NSAIDs inhibit prostaglandin production and that they relieve menstrual cramps in 65 to 100 percent of the women who use them. So even if you aren't certain why NSAIDs work, there's a pretty strong case for giving them a try.

In a double-blind study comparing aspirin and ibuprofen, 21 to 30 percent of the women taking aspirin preparations reported moderate to complete relief of pain. And 61 to 84 percent of the women taking ibuprofen reported the same. Remember that the next time you're wrapped around the heating pad and writhing in pain.

M. Yusoff Dawood, M.D., professor of reproductive endocrinology at the University of Illinois College of Medicine in Chicago, suggests that sexually active women should try to avoid all drugs, because the effects of *any* drug on an undetected pregnancy can be tragic. But if you must take a drug for your cramps, wait until your period has started, he says.

Other than that, Dr. Dawood says, choose the NSAID with the fewest side effects and the longest track record. He recommends Motrin as a first choice since it's been around the longest, works quickly, has few side effects and costs the least. Naproxen is a close runner-up; it just hasn't been around as long as Motrin.

But serious side effects have occurred with other NSAIDs, including the commonly prescribed indomethacin (Indocin). Reports indicate that almost half of all Indocin users experience side effects such as gastric irritation, headaches, dizziness and/or disorientation. Clearly, it's not the kind of thing to be taking on a regular basis as you go about your daily chores. Bathing your child, or driving your car, or washing the second-story windows would all have an extra element of risk with these side effects.

Moreover, no NSAID is appropriate if you are allergic to aspirin (except for Disalcid), have gastritis or peptic ulcers, or have any other kind of similar stomach problem, warns Dr. Dawood. And because NSAIDs are so irritating to the stomach, Dr. Dawood suggests you take them with food.

But what about over-the-counter drugs sold specifically to relieve cramps, such as Midol and Pamprin?

Well, if they work for you then they work for you. Some of these drugs are composed of aspirin plus a variety of extraneous additives such as diuretics (caffeine), muscle relaxants and antihistamines. Because of all these ingredients you might want to talk to your doctor before taking these drugs.

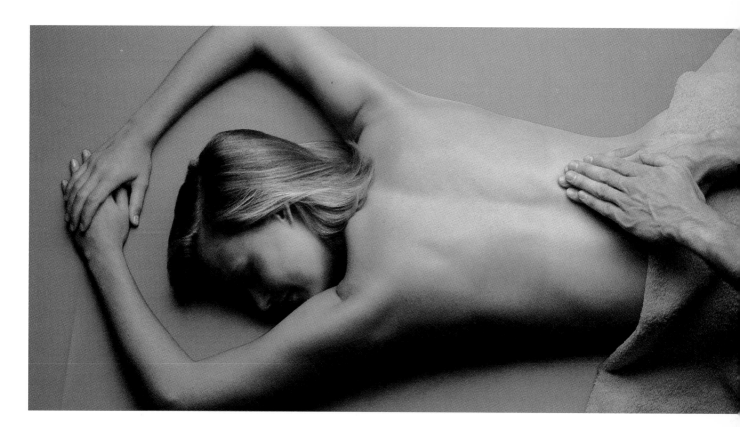

DON'T FORGET THE HUMAN ELEMENT

Along with trying the recommendations in this chapter, don't forget to also make use of the human element. This other option, suggested by William E. Whitehead, Ph.D., a research psychologist at Johns Hopkins School of Medicine, may provide effective pain relief. In a recent study, Dr. Whitehead discovered that if someone touches you when you're in pain, you'll feel better. *Really* better.

"We think that it's an innate system for mother/infant bonding," explains Dr. Whitehead—kind of a built-in mechanism that explains why Mom's old kiss-it-and-make-it-better technique really worked. Touching reduces your heart rate, explains Dr. Whitehead. And while it doesn't

reduce your pain, it does increase your ability to tolerate it.

Marvelous. Think about what a broad effect touching could have if it were consciously used to relieve pain. Not just on cramps, but on chronic pain in general. And could it be even more effective if we were "touch specific"?

What would happen, for example, if a woman with cramps asked her partner to lay a hand on her abdomen during painful contractions? What would happen if a man with a heart condition asked his wife to stroke his chest when angina put on the squeeze? Or how about one friend asking another to hold her when she's burning from carpal tunnel syndrome? Or phlebitis or ulcers or kidney stones?

The next time pain grabs you in its teeth, you should ask someone you care about for more than their sympathy. Ask for their hand.

Ah-h-h-h-h. Right there. Menstrual cramps often can be relieved by massage, says Bill Prentice, Ph.D., athletic trainer for the women's soccer team at the University of North Carolina, Chapel Hill. Next time you hurt, ask a friend to gently feel around just below the midsection of your back, 1 inch to the right of the third bony vertebra up from the base of your spine. Feel a twinge? That's the spot. Now relax and ask your friend to gently but firmly massage the spot in slow circles, using only 1 finger and continuing until the cramps stop—usually about 4 minutes.

6

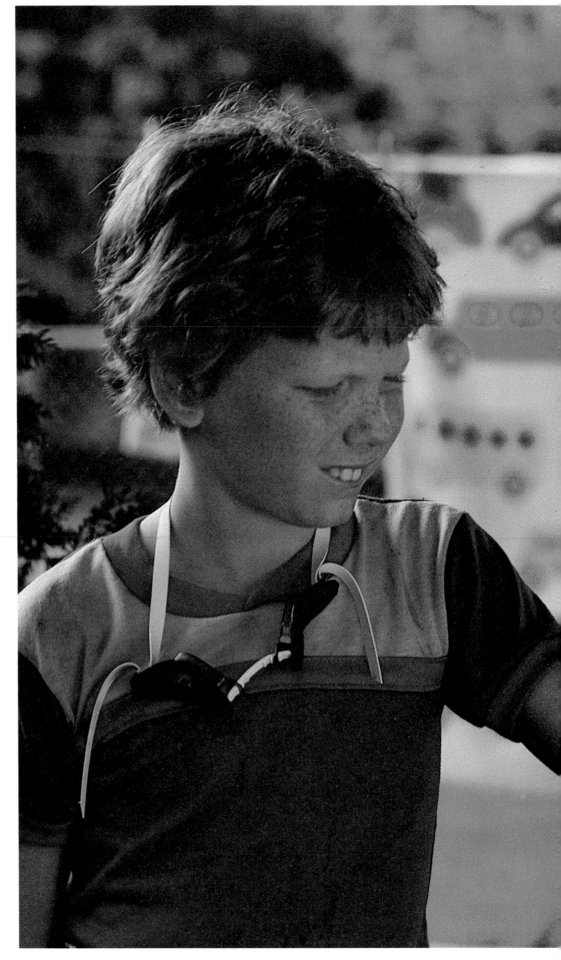

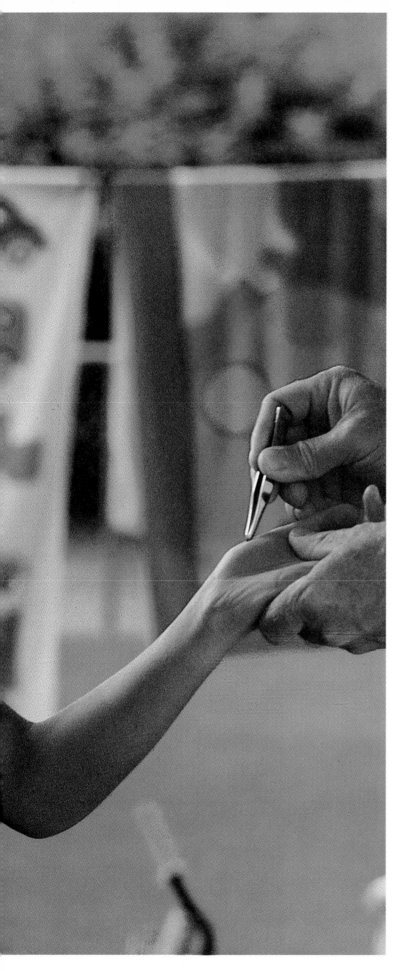

Soothing Everyday Pains

Into each life some pain must fall. Here's how to cope.

Imagine a day like this: You bang your shin on the coffee table for the umpteenth time. As you hobble to the kitchen, your son blasts out of the swinging saloon doors like ex-football coach John Madden in those beer commercials. The left panel flattens your nose while the right bites a chip off your front tooth.

In the kitchen, you open the oven to check the progress of a sizzling sirloin. Instantly, a tiny explosion launches a flaming comet of fat onto your forearm. You jerk your hand up in agony— right into the broiler heating element.

You rush outside for respite. A wasp nesting under your porch decides to protect her family by digging a poison-laden stinger deep into your neck.

You tumble to the grass. A cockroach crawls into your right ear and starts doing the rumba. A gnat flies into your left ear and begins singing "Mack the Knife."

You crawl to the empty lot next door and get a rusty nail in your foot, a thorn in your side, a splinter in your finger and a dirt speck of biblical proportions in your eye.

Running back to your property, your foot catches in a groundhog hole. The foot holds, but the rest of you hits the turf. That clever demonstration of nimbleness results in a stubbed toe, a sprained ankle, a twisted knee and a pulled muscle in your groin. Despite that, you have no trouble getting up—the frenzied fire ants whose hill you flattened see to that.

Though it's doubtful anyone other than Jerry Lewis ever hit such a nightmarish streak, chances are you will suffer many if not all of these everyday pains at some time in your life. One at a time.

To help prepare you for these minor emergencies, we've targeted the most common ones, then consulted some of the best medical specialists in the nation for pain-relieving solutions.

CURSED CANKERS

Tiny white circles of fire, they burn the mouth's interior, making eating, drinking and sometimes talking an agonizing experience. They afflict 80 percent of us, and so far have laughed at medical science. As the old joke goes, most doctors feel that if you treat them, they'll go away in seven days. Leave them alone and they'll last a week.

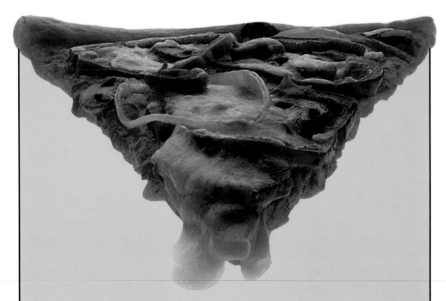

Pizza Pain

As soon as the delivery man is out the door you take a big bite of that wedge-shaped, tomato-sauce-and-cheese-covered slice and instantly discover that lack of patience may make you a patient. The tasty, melted mozzarella cheese is actually a savage sheet of gooey fire. It clutches the defenseless roof of your mouth and transfers the full fury of its 450 degrees. Culinary ecstasy soon turns to agony. Doctors have dubbed this painful burn pizza palate. Mark L. Dembert, M.D., of the U.S. Navy Medical Corps, and Halley S. Faust, M.D., of Lexington, Kentucky, offer these tips for relief from pizza palate: Ask your doctor or dentist for a lidocaine anesthetic mouthwash, and rinse with it; suck on over-the-counter lozenges and cough drops that contain soothing benzocaine. To avoid aggravating the area, stick to an all-liquid diet for 2 days, then soft foods for 2 more. Steer clear of crusty foods and hot foods for a week.

Doctors say cankers are almost as difficult to diagnose as to cure. Hueston C. King, M.D., an otolaryngologist (ear, nose and throat specialist) from Venice, Florida, explains, "One theory is that the true canker sore is a herpes simplex virus, the same virus that causes fever blisters (also known as cold sores). The confusion is that a very similar problem can result from aphthous ulcers, which are not caused by the herpes virus.

"How do you know what you have? Good question," he says. "A lot of us doctors can't tell the difference. As far as getting rid of them goes, it doesn't really matter. There is really no good treatment for either one.

"But there are ways to fight the pain," according to Dr. King. "Dabbing vinegar on the sores can help, or anything that makes you pucker. A commercial peroxide rinse (Gly-Oxide) can ease pain."

According to medical experts, peroxide rinses can be used up to four times a day—after each meal and at bedtime. Place several drops on the sores, wait 2 or 3 minutes, then spit. Another method is to put about ten drops on the tongue, mix it with saliva, swish it around for several minutes, then spit. Do not rinse. Avoid getting the rinses in your eyes. If an amount exceeding recommended dosage is accidentally swallowed, seek immediate medical assistance or contact a poison control center.

"You can touch the sore with a styptic pencil to ease pain," Dr. King adds. "A dab of alum on a cotton swab sometimes works. For really bad cases, a smallpox vaccine works about 25 percent of the time.

"As for lysine (an amino acid widely promoted as a herpes cure), one person will say it works, the next ten will say it doesn't. Obviously, we need more research," he says.

Past research on the controversial lysine subject includes a study by Richard S. Griffith, M.D., of the Indiana University School of Medicine, in which 45 cold sore sufferers were given from 312 to 1,200 milligrams of lysine daily. For most, pain was reported to disappear overnight and healing was hastened. Continued lysine supplements were said to prevent further sores.

The exact dosage of lysine was further defined in a subsequent study by four doctors at the Mayo Clinic, Rochester, Minnesota. Studying 47 patients, they determined that a dose of 624 milligrams a day was not effective, but increasing the dose to 1,248 milligrams showed evidence of decreasing the recurrence rate of herpes simplex attacks.

However, a study performed at the University of Miami School of Medicine concluded that daily doses of 1,200 milligrams of lysine had, for most people, no effect whatsoever on herpes.

While researchers debate, those bothered by canker sores may want to try lysine to see if it helps.

Also try to avoid stress, says Dr. King. Sunburn, fever, antibiotics, food allergies, acidic foods, dehydration, exhaustion or "anything that puts a severe stress on the body's system" can bring them on.

Fever blisters, which form on the outside of the lips, may have the same cause and can be treated in a manner similar to that for cankers, according to Dr. King.

While treating the sores topically and avoiding stress, it's also wise to monitor your nutrition. A study of 330 canker sufferers by doctors in Glasgow, Scotland, showed that 14 percent had nutritional deficiencies of either iron, folate, vitamin B_{12} or all three. When the patients were treated with supplements, the cankers were eliminated or greatly reduced.

You also may want to forgo the filberts. Harold C. Fishman, M.D., of Los Angeles, found that a whopping 80 percent of his canker-suffering patients over a 30-year period had one common link—they were nut lovers. This would support studies that say a disturbed arginine/lysine balance may cause cankers, since nuts (and chocolate) are high in arginine, an amino acid.

Your doctor should be able to advise you about the latest research concerning these and other treatments.

SOOTHING SCRATCHY THROATS

"For sore throats, warm salt water gargles and plenty of antiseptic loz-enges fight the pain," Dr. King says. "Vitamin C has been observed to help, but there's no scientific proof. In reasonable amounts, it can't hurt.

"If it's a minor sore throat with no fever and lasts less than three days, you probably don't need to go to a doctor," he says. "If you have a fever or the pain lasts longer than three days, see a doctor.

"If the tonsils are inflamed, painkillers like acetaminophen [Datril, Tylenol] or aspirin can help," according to Dr. King. "However, if you're scheduled for surgery, you should not take aspirin a week prior to an operation, because it hinders blood clotting. Acetaminophen has no negative effect."

TORMENTING TOOTHACHES

"Sex!" proclaims Richard Kaufman, D.D.S., high-spirited orthodontist from Oceanside, New York. "That's the best toothache cure of all. I've never known anyone to complain of a toothache while having sex!"

Unfortunately, even the most insatiable among us can divert the mind with sex for only so long. Toothaches tend to have more stamina.

"Clove oil eases toothache pain," Dr. Kaufman was persuaded to add. "Apply it directly to the tooth. If you have pain for longer than a few hours, go to the dentist."

The FDA agrees that clove oil does the trick. In a report of 12 active ingredients in common toothache remedies, the government regulation agency found that clove oil was the only one that worked.

"If a filling pops out, reach for the clove oil again," Dr. Kaufman says. (But keep the bottle out of reach of your children. Like a lot of other substances, this oil is poisonous in very big doses.) "You can also roll a piece of cotton in a tiny ball and gently plug the hole until you can see your dentist, which should be as soon as possible. This temporary measure will keep food from getting in and increasing the pain. I don't recommend patients treating themselves with commercial fillings. You could pack it too high and damage the opposing tooth.

"If it's a large filling, or an

Mouth Pain Relief?

The American Dental Association's (ADA) Council on Dental Therapeutics lists as acceptable a number of commercial pastes, gels and liquids that may relieve the pain of cankers and cold sores. The ingredients to look for are benzocaine and lidocaine. However, the ADA cautions that they provide only temporary relief of symptoms and do not treat the cause.

The only way to treat the cause, says the ADA, and thus the pain (and *only* with cold sores caused by herpes virus) is with acyclovir, a prescription drug sold under the brand name Zovirax. Ask your doctor about this drug.

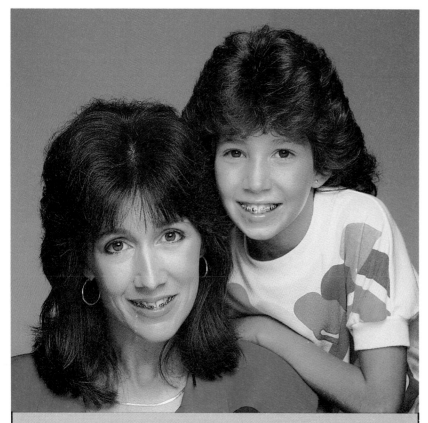

Bracing for the Pain

"Psssst," one teenager says, motioning to another. "Wanna buy a wax strip? Fifty cents." Exaggerated, yes. But not too far-fetched. The wax strips are what orthodontists give people to protect their mouths from the rough edges of braces. That relief makes them a valuable commodity in high school hallways. "To avoid postpubescent profiteers, your orthodontist can fit you with a permanent, protective piece of soft plastic shaped like a U," says Richard Kaufman, D.D.S., of Oceanside, New York. "Aspirin can help relieve the pain if it gets bad. To prevent pain, oral hygiene is vital. Special soft toothbrushes are available, and the water spray devices are good. Gly-Oxide and Brace-Aid cleaning liquids also help. A circular electric toothbrush called a Rota-dent, available through most dentists, has different brushes specifically recommended for brace wearers."

For those who suffer the greatest pain when looking in the mirror, Dr. Kaufman says there are now "invisible" braces that are affixed on the inside of the teeth. The trouble is, they cost twice as much, cause more irritation and are less comfortable. Such is the price of vanity.

exposed nerve results in severe pain, I would call a dentist immediately," he adds.

"If you chip or break a tooth, keep your mouth closed and breathe through your nose," Dr. Kaufman advises. "Air striking the nerve causes chilling pain. Stay away from any hot or cold things. Covering the tooth with clove oil can help, but you must see your dentist as soon as possible."

Once you're at the dentist, you may be pleasantly surprised to find that your treatment is painless. Eva J. Mertz-Fairhurst, D.D.S., associate professor in the department of restorative dentistry at the Medical College of Georgia in Augusta, discovered in a seven-year study of 382 children that she was able to stifle the spread of cavities without using the hated drill! Instead, Dr. Mertz-Fairhurst covered the tooth with a clear plastic sealant. Consult your dentist for an update on these and other pain-free techniques.

HANDS OFF YOUR EARS

"Earaches are one thing you don't treat off-the-cuff. You only get two ears to a customer. If you have any pain at all don't use a self-applied home remedy—go see a doctor," says Dr. King.

"I don't recommend sticking *anything* in your ear. It's just too risky," he says.

"Stay out of the ear," agrees Lewis Goldfrank, M.D., director of emergency medical services at New York's Bellevue Hospital. "If you have pain and can't immediately get to a doctor, take some aspirin or acetaminophen, but that's it."

With these admonishments firmly in mind, there are things you can do externally to combat ear irritations.

Major Trauma. If you think you have a major problem like a ruptured eardrum, the American Medical Association (AMA) suggests easing the pain prior to going to the doctor by covering the ear with an electric heating pad set on low.

Airplane Pain. Remember Dumbo? The chubby little elephant used his ears to fly. Ironically, flying and ears are actually painful enemies. Air pressure is the instigator.

"Just before and during descent of the airplane, swallow frequently," says Stanley N. Farb, M.D., an otolaryngologist from Philadelphia. If that doesn't help, Dr. Farb suggests pinching your nose shut as you swallow, or chewing gum.

Clogged Ears. For ears stuffed up by a cold or flu, Donald Vickery, M.D., of Reston, Virginia, says a vaporizer or steamy shower can gently bring soothing moisture into the ear.

Swimmers' Ear. A little moisture may help the ear, but a lot can hurt it. Infections often wash into a swimmer's ears along with the chlorine. If you experience postpool pain, off to the doctor you go. He'll probably prescribe antibiotics. To help prevent swimmer's ear, doctors recommend putting four or five drops of isopropyl alcohol (70%) into each ear when you finish your swim. Divers should remember that our sound receptors have the same trouble below the surface as they do high above—changes in pressure. Learn how to handle it from both your doctor and a professional diving instructor.

Bugs and Blocks. Bugs find the human ear to be a warm, cozy place to hang out. If your ear canal becomes a housing project, don't try to evict the tenant with a poke or a prod. Instead, try leaning your head over to see if the critter falls out. If it doesn't, slip a drop of olive oil into the ear. The oil may kill it, but it also may leave you with a dead bug in your ear. If this happens, gently syringe the ear with water to flush it out. If it still won't vacate, let a doctor serve the eviction notice.

Itching Ears. Hair products are generally the villain. Watch out for the itchy six—hair spray, permanent wave lotion, dyes, perfumes, shampoo and mousses. If you notice a rash or itch after using any of these products, switch brands.

THE AGONY OF DE FEET

Which exerts more weight per square inch, a loaded, 18-wheel tractor-trailer or a 115-pound woman in high

Blackboard Pain

For many, the most horrifying scene in the movie *Jaws* wasn't when the shark crunched somebody; it was when the salty old sea captain clawed his fingernails across a blackboard to get the attention of the noisy city commissioners. Scientists and doctors admit the sound irritates us, but why?

Major John H. Elmore, an audiologist who is chief of the Air Force's Hearing Conservation Data Registry, offers a theory. "It's learned behavior, a perceived pain. You could listen to that sound all day without suffering any damage to the internal ear structures. It may be extremely annoying, and in turn cause tension and negative chemical reactions in the body, but it's not hurting your ears."

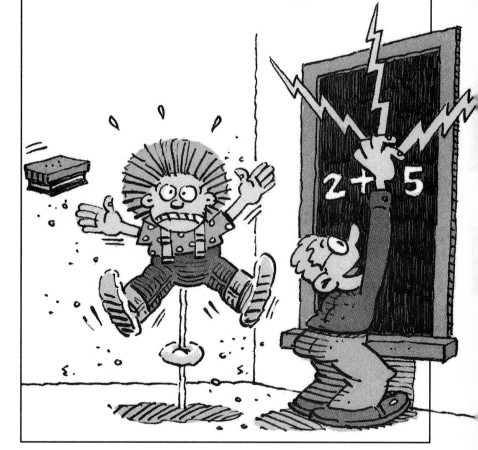

heels? Believe it or not, they're the same, each handling 65 pounds per square inch. Just one look at the cracks and craters in the average highway gives a vivid indication of the similar pounding your feet take. And where there's pounding, there's usually pain.

Fortunately, where there's pain, you'll generally find a podiatrist ready to conquer it. Here are some self-help hints foot specialists suggest to help you get a foot up on foot pain.

Corns. "Soaking your feet in a pan of warm water with ½ to 1 cup of Epsom salt will help ease the pain." says Dennis Augustine, D.P.M., direc-tor of the Park Avenue Foot Clinic in San Jose, California. "You can also pour in ½ cup of white vinegar to take the sting and soreness out.

Pain-Relieving Trio for Flat Feet

Painful flat feet? Dennis F. Augustine, D.P.M., of San Jose, California, says a rolling pin, a massage and a pan of warm water can get you hopping. "A rolling pin is good in terms of building up arch muscles. Just sit down, put your foot over the pin and roll forward and backward 50 times one way, 50 times the other. A second method is to gently massage the foot to relax it, stimulate circulation and bring nutrition to the muscles. The best way is to start with the heel, using the thumbs to massage. Move to the arch, then gently caress the ball of the foot. Advance to each individual toe, softly pulling and stroking them. Use some form of oil, cream or petroleum jelly [see also "How to Give a Foot Massage" on pages 108-109]. Finally, a warm water and Epsom salt soak is always a winner. Those little home whirlpool units are an added boost."

"For a top corn, put some moleskin (available at most drugstores) over the area. For a softer corn in between the toes, secure some lamb's wool around it for a cushion," he recommends.

For serious corn pain, Dr. Augustine suggests taking aspirin or an ibuprofen-based painkiller such as Motrin. "Stay away from commercial acid plasters or pads with chemicals that are supposed to burn the corn off. These may harm the surrounding skin. If the corn is bad, your podiatrist can relieve the pain with a minor, painless surgical procedure."

Calluses. Elizabeth Roberts, D.P.M., of New York, author of *On Your Feet*, says you can treat calluses the same way as corns, with a few exceptions.

"I prefer a spot pad over moleskin because I disapprove of putting any stickiness over an area that is irritated. A dressing of sterile gauze is good," she says. "When you remove any dressing, be sure you ease it in a slow, slow motion toward the heel to avoid tearing skin. Remove the dressing when bathing or sleeping to maintain skin tone."

Bunions. "These are tougher," Dr. Augustine explains. "They usually have to be removed. In the meantime, you can wear a wider shoe, pad the area to take the pressure off, soak your foot and take aspirin."

Cracked, Dry Feet. "Creams relieve the pain here," Dr. Augustine advises. "Vitamin A or E creams or aloe vera are quite effective. Rub them on your feet two to three times a day, especially in the morning. Joggers or people on their feet all day should wear a thin, silk sock under a second, more absorbent cotton sock.

Stubbed Toes. "Apply ice for the first 24 hours on and off, and take two aspirin every 4 to 6 hours. After the first day, change to a warm soak with ½ cup of vinegar in 2 quarts of water and a cup of Epsom salt. If the pain doesn't subside in a few days, see your doctor," says Dr. Augustine.

Athlete's Foot. "The itch can become pain if left untreated. There are plenty of readily available over-the-

counter medications. These usually work. If the condition doesn't respond in a week, or the fungus gets into your nails, see a podiatrist," Dr. Augustine advises.

Ingrown Nails. "If the nail is just beginning to cut into the flesh, pack a little cotton into the nail groove between the edge of the nail and the flesh. Do not go into the nail grooves with anything else!" Dr. Roberts warns. "If the pain is severe, you should see a podiatrist.

"To avoid ingrown nails, cut your nails straight across. Don't cut the corners. If that rips your socks,

Feet on the Beat

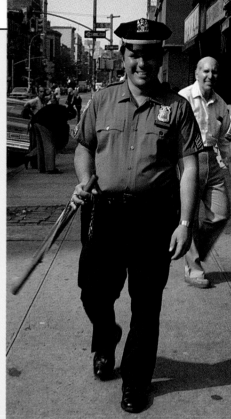

On the mean street beat, they're the heat. And their feet gotta stay sweet. That sums up life in New York City's Community Patrol Program, a squad of officers who keep the peace on the Lower East Side by walking the beat. Obviously, painful feet can be a problem. So foot care is vital. "The first thing is a good shoe," says Sgt. Dean Rasinya. "I prefer a good lace shoe, not a loafer. They are more comfortable and provide more support. In summer, I wear a thin sock to let the air in. In winter, I slip on a nylon sock inside for insulation, covered with a wool sock for warmth. I use a foot powder all year. I put it in the sock itself and in the shoe, and sprinkle it between my toes. The foot powders fight perspiration and prickly heat. Sometimes I change shoes, especially on the 4:00 P.M. to midnight shift. I really get beat, and changing my shoes and socks refreshes me. Washing the feet also refreshes them. Since I take good care of my feet, I don't need to soak them much, and I don't have corns or bunions. If you maintain good hygiene and wear a good shoe, you've got foot pain beat."

use an emery board to file the edges down," she advises.

While home remedies can ease foot pain, Dr. Roberts puts her foot down when it comes to relying on them.

"Corns, calluses, ingrown nails—they are all an indication of a more fundamental problem," she warns. "If you cure the pain and forget about the basic condition, the problem will grow worse. If you walk differently to avoid the pain, you could develop leg, knee, hip or low back pain. You have to see a podiatrist to find out why you have these problems."

EASING CHILDREN'S PAIN

If your kids play any sport, organized or not, you know that minor injuries are inevitable. Bert M. Franks, M.D., a Texas pediatrician who specializes in sports medicine, says children need special care for all their hurts.

Bad References

Doctors call it referred pain, meaning one area of the body is injured or diseased but the pain is someplace else. This is because many areas of the body are connected to the same nerve system funneling into the spinal cord. Damage to the diaphragm, lungs or heart, for example, is often felt in the shoulder. A diseased pancreas or gallbladder frequently refers pain to a point between the shoulder blades. A heart attack or angina sometimes sends pain to the arm.

Ironically, one of the most commonly touted examples of referred pain is technically a misconception. This is ye ol' funny bone sensation. According to Carol A. Warfield, M.D., director of the pain management unit at Beth Israel Hospital, Boston, the tingling felt in your fingers when you bang your elbow is the normal process of the signal temporarily shooting down the ulnar nerve. The elbow still hurts and hasn't really passed the buck. The same sensation can happen along the sciatic nerve, which extends from the back to the toes.

"You're dealing with a low pain threshold combined with high fear," he explains. "Parents must reassure the injured child that he will be okay. Parents must be as calm as possible. You can't panic. That panics the child.

"If it's a cut, the first thing is to stop the bleeding. Blood frightens the child and parents as well. Put pressure on the cut with cloth, tissue or gauze and hold it down 15 minutes without looking at it. If it continues to bleed, see a doctor. If the child is in pain, put some ice in a cloth and place it over the cut for 20 to 30 minutes while you are riding to the doctor," he advises.

"For bruises, ice in a plastic bag relieves pain and slows down bleeding, plus it reassures the child that the parent is making it better.

"As for cuts, scrapes and grass burns, I personally don't believe in topical antipain medications," says Dr. Franks. "Cleaning the wound with soap and water, applying a light coat of antibiotic ointment and putting on a dressing will do. Then let them go back out and play. That will divert their minds from the pain. I believe in letting children set their own pace. They don't need to be overprotected. If it's a great big scrape, remind them to stay out of the dirt.

"A broken arm or leg obviously needs medical attention as soon as possible. You can relieve the immediate pain with ice, immobilization and elevating the limb above the level of the heart. Put an ice bag on the broken limb, hold it in a pillow, or construct a sling. You can use a magazine or stick for a splint," he says.

MINISICKNESSES

For the more routine illnesses children pick up in the course of turning into adults, pediatrician Paul Dunn, M.D., and his wife Kathryn, a nutritional consultant—parents of ten children—offer these tips from their Oak Park, Illinois, medical practice.

Sore Throats. "An older child can gargle with salt water to relieve minor infections," Dr. Dunn says. "Younger children can take acetaminophen drops (Tylenol, Datril). Throat lozenges can provide some relief. Any sore throat that lasts longer than two days or is accompanied by a cold, coughing, fever, vomiting or diarrhea should be treated by a doctor," he says.

Earaches. "Be careful here. If it's minor, some ear drops and warm compresses might ease the pain. Decongestants or nose drops (in the nose, of course) may also help. Tylenol is effective. If the child slows down, is not eating or shows any other ill signs, take him or her to a doctor immediately," Dr. Dunn stresses.

Growing Pains. These pains do not come from growing. "Children have pain from activity and muscle strains, not from the act of growing," Dr. Dunn says. "It doesn't hurt for cells to multiply. Muscle pain, for example, shouldn't be ignored. The pain is real. Sitting in a warm tub can provide some real relief. The parent can gently massage the area that hurts. Mildly exercising a sore muscle may also help. If the pain persists for two days or more, see a doctor."

Flus, Colds, Fevers. "You must treat these symptomatically, with specific treatments for the ears, throat and muscles as we have mentioned," Dr. Dunn advises. "Use acetaminophen for pain, and give the sick child lots of fluids. Additional vitamin C is also indicated, perhaps 150 to 200 milligrams. If the illness persists for more than two days or becomes serious, see your doctor."

BUNDLES OF PAIN

Helping babies over their aches and pains is quite a bit harder than helping older children. Why? Because they can't talk. Parents are often left wringing their hands, wondering just *what* hurts the baby, and how intense the pain is. "Parents often can distinguish between their babies' cries for hunger, a diaper change or pain, but they may also overreact or underreact. I didn't use antibiotics and painkillers much with my own kids, but I was there to diagnose the seriousness.

It's best to let your doctor handle it," Dr. Dunn says.

"For routine teething, a teething ring can give temporary reliief. Some of the commercial gels and creams may work, but I never use them. I prefer some acetaminophen drops. Colic is another common illness, but I don't favor home treatment," he says. "Sometimes it's caused by a food intolerence or a sensitivity to cow's milk and switching the formula can help. The best thing is to call your doctor. You shouldn't take a chance with a baby."

HOME REMEDIES

A former teacher of anatomy and physiology at Charity Hospital School of Nursing in New Orleans, Mrs. Dunn is a proponent of home remedies. Here's what she suggests for various ailments.

"When a baby is teething, there is a general depression of his overall immune system. This is the time to give the baby supplementary vitamin C to protect it. Also, when they are having their routine immunization shots, give them extra vitamin C," she says.

"For earaches, we've found that in some cases, an allergy to cow's milk is the problem," Dr. Dunn interjects. "Milk sensitivity may increase mucus and can also depress the white blood cell count. This can be a significant factor in recurring earaches. We see a lot of this in our practice. Have your doctor perform an allergy test. If it turns up positive for milk, eliminating *all* milk products for a period of six months and reintroducing only small amounts carefully can help."

"Skin problems, cuts, scratches and scrapes can be soothed with creams containing vitamins A and E, and taking vitamin C. Burns are also helped by aloe vera," Mrs. Dunn continues.

BURN TREATMENTS— A GREASY DILEMMA

Raging volcanoes, bubbling hot springs and sun-scorched rocks taught our ancestors about the searing pain of burns. Progress has given us fire, electricity and radiation—all new, more ingenious ways of burning holes in our hides.

Fortunately, doctors say new treatments combined with age-old remedies can counter these perils of modern society. Which isn't to say there haven't been disagreements. Most concern the use of grease-based substances.

"The essence of the grease controversy is that the skin will heal more quickly and feel better if covered, but grease increases the chance of infection to a small extent," says Karl Kramer, M.D., a clinical professor of dermatology at the University of Miami School of Medicine. "I feel if the burn doesn't break the skin, then just use cold water. If the skin is broken, I have no problems with using grease. I use grease in the form of an antibiotic cream containing silver sulfadiazine to avoid infection."

A study by a team of researchers headed by Charles L. Fox, Jr., M.D., of New York, concluded that zinc sulfadiazine is also an effective antibiotic cream to use on burns.

A study performed by A. G. Shulman, M.D., of Los Angeles, on 150 burn patients suffering from chemical, heat or electrical burns concluded that immediate immersion

in cold water was able to immediately reduce pain, reduce total treatment time and burn severity by two-thirds and reduce infection. Cold water immersion also reduces damage to the skin and in some cases prevents blistering. The study found that effectiveness may depend upon how soon you get the burned area under cold water. Even 10 minutes can make a difference between minor redness and a nasty skin blister. The study also recommended keeping the burned area submerged for 30 minutes to 2 hours, or until there is no pain when it is taken out of the cold water.

Updating his study, Dr. Shulman offers these clarifications.

"Direct ice is not to be used, nor is cold running water. Both are painful. I suggest immersion in what I call comfortably cold water. There is no specific temperature range because everybody is different. The patient must be the judge, using freedom from pain as a guide to the correct temperature. While the burned area is being treated under cold water—or with a cold, wet washcloth if the area cannot be easily submerged—the rest of the body should be warmed with blankets, hot water bottles, sweaters or whatever. This will make it easier for the patient to tolerate the

Kitchen Burners

"Hour Magazine" resident chef Laurie Burrows Grad knows the dangers that lurk in a kitchen. Here's her advice on avoiding burns.

- Use the mitts that your hand slides into, not flimsy potholders. And never grab a hot handle with a wet towel.
- Avoid cooking in disposable foil pans. They can overheat and cause the grease to ignite.
- If you deep fry, use a wok set tightly in a ring. It's deep, doesn't splatter and is hard to knock over.
- Keep some aloe vera plants in the kitchen. If you get burned, rub on some of the juice.

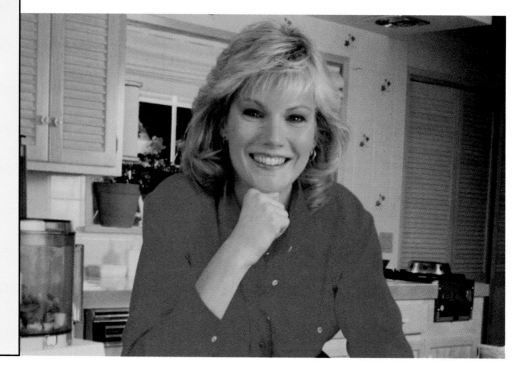

cold over the burned area. People often say 'I'm too cold' and give up," he says. "Warming the unburned part takes care of that."

Remember, this technique is to be used only for superficial burns over a small area. "And never immerse the entire body in ice water. That can be dangerous, even fatal," Dr. Shulman warns.

If water is good, what's bad?

"What you should never use on a burn is iodine or Mercurochrome. They are toxic and can burn the patient and increase the pain," warns Richard Knutson, M.D., an orthopedic surgeon at the Delta Medical Center in Greenville, Mississippi.

Here are some additional tips from Dr. Knutson for specific burns.

Fire. "Immediately immerse or place an ice pack on the burned area for ½ hour to 45 minutes. For large burns, or if you continue to swell after the burn, go to a doctor. If you're severely burned, stay calm. Go to the refrigerator and take some cold water, ice cubes, a veal roast or whatever's cold and place it on the area. Call someone to come help you. Don't rush around. If your clothes are stuck to your skin, don't worry. Let a doctor remove them," he advises.

Scalding Water. "If you spill scalding water on yourself, immediately remove any clothing from the areas where the water has soaked. Tight-fitting wool or polyester clothing, especially socks and pants, hold the heat and increase the damage. Ice packs or cold water are the best treatments," says Dr. Knutson.

Cooking Oils, Grease. "These burns are more devastating because the temperature of these liquids is so high. (Water boils at 212°F; heated oil can reach 400° to 500°.) The time factor here is vital. Rip off the soaked clothes instantly. Treat the pain the same way as burns caused by hot water," Dr. Knutson says.

Tar, Polypropylene Cord. "These melted substances can be removed painlessly with WD 40 spray, the gun-cleaning solvent available in most drug and hardware stores. Polypropylene cords are used as ropes and ties

by boaters and skiers and are routinely burned to secure frayed ends. The melting polypropylene often drops on the hand or leg, causing considerable pain," Dr. Knutson explains. "Spraying the WD 40 oil will cause the melted substance to drip off. Pine oil disinfectant or turpentine are alternatives, although they may sting a bit at first."

Sunburn. "Any of the topical commercial sprays are soothing. Ice and cold showers also will help. Aloe vera relieves the swelling and eases the pain quickly. I use that myself," Dr. Knutson remarks. "You should also be extremely careful to replenish electrolytes (ion conductors that regulate fluid and acid balance, mainly sodium, potassium, calcium, magnesium and chloride) and lost water by drinking fluids," he says.

Friction Burns. "Rope burns can be very dangerous because they dig deep. Ice, grease and sugar are best for pain relief. If you have swelling and/or increasing pain, go to a doctor."

PAIN IN PARADISE

Escape the kitchen and the danger of burns and venture into the great outdoors. Blue skies. Lush forests. Pristine lakes. Soft grass. Gentle breezes. Fragrant flowers.

Flowers? Thorns. Bees. Allergies. Rashes.

Forests? Spiders. Splinters. Poison ivy. Ticks. Fire ants. Cuts. Scratches.

Lakes? Mosquitoes. Snapping turtles. Submerged, sharp objects teeming with germs.

Sometime, somewhere, somebody must have fooled Mother Nature, because the old gal has been sticking it to us, painfully, ever since. Whether you hunt, fish, camp, hike, sail, ski or just stroll through a park, the Boy Scout motto "Be Prepared" should be foremost in mind.

"The main thing to do with any injuries of the skin is to disinfect," says Rodney Basler, M.D., a Lincoln, Nebraska, dermatologist who's familiar with outdoor injuries. "If you can keep the bacteria out of the wounds, you can minimize the pain. Rubbing

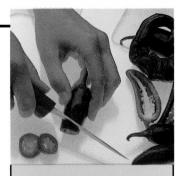

Chili Heat

Those familiar with Szechuan and Mexican foods know that the oils in hot peppers can cause your hands to sizzle, as well as your mouth. If your hands burn after cutting up hot peppers, here's a tip from cooks in Texas and Mexico: Soak your hot hands in vinegar for a few minutes. To avoid the pain altogether, wear gloves when you slice. And don't scratch your eyes and nose, or you'll spread the burning oil.

The Troublesome Knee

The human knee wasn't designed to withstand extreme punishment. This limitation caused the cloud that rained on the careers of Joe Namath, Gale Sayers, Mickey Mantle, Dick Butkus, Bubba Smith and hundreds of other athletes. Recent advances in microscopic surgery were all that saved Olympic gold medal gymnast Mary Lou Retton and marathoner Joan Benoit Samuelson from a similar fate.

Yet knee injuries don't savage just the famous. Thomas F. Griffin, Jr., M.D., a sports medicine expert from Douglas, Arizona, says weekend athletes who suffer severe pain, hear a popping noise or tear, or develop an unstable knee should seek immediate medical treatment. If your knee hurts when you bear weight or hurts for more than three days, see your doctor. For minor twists and sprains, Dr. Griffin suggests using a common pro football technique. Wrap the knee once with a long Ace bandage. Put ice over the first bandage layer, then finish by wrapping over the ice to secure it to the knee. Elevating the knee will also comfort it. Aspirin or ibuprofen can reduce inflammation and deflate lingering pain. Dr. Griffin warns, however, that using drugs to dull the pain without seeing a doctor may result in further damage.

To avoid knee trouble in the first place, Stanley G. Newell, M.D., a podiatrist from Seattle, offers these tips to prevent common knee injuries.
- Wear the proper shoes for individual sports and check for uneven wear.
- Make sure your shoes and supports fit properly.
- Increase your workout time or jogging mileage no more than 10 percent every other week.
- Shorten your strides when running downhill.
- If you change from a hard to soft or soft to hard playing or running surface, says Dr. Newell, divide your workouts between them the first few weeks to give your body time to adjust to the change.

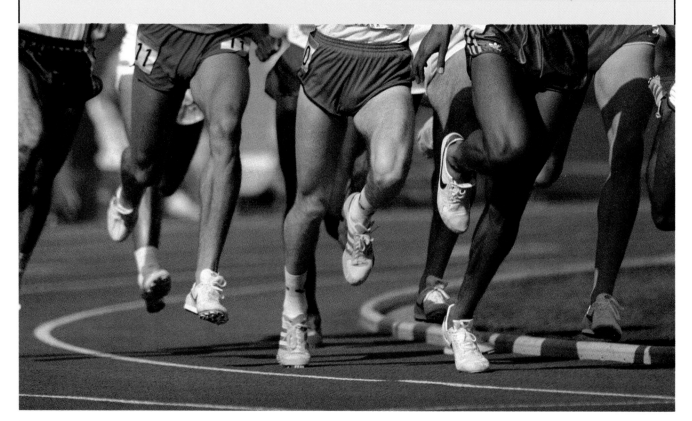

realm of possible injuries—an arena thousands enter each day. The growing emphasis on health and vigor has induced us to dust off our racquets, clubs, bats and balls and head out to the hardwood courts, lanes, links, diamonds, jogging trails, bicycle paths and grass or artificially turfed fields.

For the majority, the rewards are toned, invigorated bodies, rejuvenated cardiovascular systems and relief from stress. However, the price can be sprains, twists, shinsplints, pulls, cramps and a host of other sports-related injuries.

"In assessing sports-related pain, consider when it occurs in relation to the activity," advises David Apple, Jr., M.D., team physician for the Atlanta Hawks NBA basketball team. "The least serious pain is that which occurs after the activity but disappears within 24 hours. The next serious is pain which is present when you start your activity but disappears as the activity continues. The most serious is pain which grows worse with activity. Usually this requires medical attention."

Thomas F. Griffin, Jr., M.D., medical director of the Douglas Clinic in Douglas, Arizona, and a specialist in sports medicine, offers these tips on how to handle the agonies of both victory and defeat.

Sprains. "Place ice in a plastic bag or towel and put it on the sprained area, and try to elevate the injury above the heart. These measures will reduce pain and swelling. A good over-the-counter pain reliever is ibuprofen [Advil, Nuprin]. In my experience, this relieves the pain, inflammation and swelling better than aspirin," he says.

"You shouldn't soak sprains in warm water because that increases the blood flow and may induce a throbbing pain and additional swelling," Dr. Griffin advises. "If you have some stiffness two to three days after the injury, you can then soak it briefly to loosen it up. Otherwise, keep it high and dry.

"A good rule is never to apply heat in the first 48 hours after an injury," agrees Dr. Apple. "Heat is mainly useful to loosen stiff joints and make the area feel better."

Regarding specific sprains, the

doctors say to watch out for wrists.

"Wrist sprains can be the most dangerous," says Dr. Griffin. "If the pain lasts more than 48 hours, see a doctor, because the small wrist bones can disintegrate and cause a permanent dysfunction of the hand.

"For knees and ankles, the pain should subside in three days. If not, see your doctor. If you feel pain when bearing weight after 24 hours, I would see a doctor. If you hear a popping or ripping or become unstable on the knee or ankle, see a doctor immediately," he warns.

Muscle Cramps. "Reach for the calcium and potassium," says Dr. Griffin. "Cramps are usually caused by electrolyte disturbances. Chicken soup is wonderful, particularly if you boil the bones. Drinking tonic or quinine water also provides the nutrients that both ease the pain and quiet muscle spasms. (This advice doesn't apply to pregnant women: Drinking very large doses of quinine water can cause uterine contractions that may lead to miscarriage.) Sardines, milk and salmon (with bones) are other sources of calcium and potassium. You can usually gain relief from the pain within an hour after eating or drinking these things.

"Topically, stretching the muscle in the opposite direction can be relieving. If the cramp is in the foot, pull up your toes," he says. "If a major cramp lasts longer than ½ hour or severely limits your ability to function, or if you have multiple cramps over a period of a week, see a doctor."

Muscle Pulls. "Ice and elevation will soothe the pain of minor pulls. If the pain interferes with sleep, try one or two 500-milligram tryptophan tablets, a natural amino acid that relieves pain and induces sleep," Dr. Griffin explains. "But don't rest too much. If you become inactive, a muscle pull can 'stove up.' That's cowboy talk for stiffening and tightening up. Stay active, but make sure you have a good warm-up period."

"This is an important but often forgotten step," agrees Dr. Apple. "Muscles can become tight and weakened after an injury. Resuming normal workouts without doing stretching

When to Quit

Pro jocks gain respect and adulation for "playing with pain." But you'll get nothing but an aggravated injury. The pros are constantly under medical supervision; you aren't. To avoid serious injury, be wary of any pain in the knee, hip and ankle joints. If they hurt, rest for a few days until pain subsides. If pain strikes while you're playing, stop and walk until it disappears. If it persists, call it a day and ice the area down at home. Any pain that lasts more than 2 days should be treated by a doctor.

and strengthening exercises often will lead to relapse or reinjury."

"If you see any surface defects such as a dip or depression in the muscle," continues Dr. Griffin, "if you have pain when bearing weight or the pain lasts longer than three days, see a doctor."

Shinsplints. "Ice, elevation and ibuprofen are the painkillers here. Stop doing whatever caused the problem for at least two weeks, and sometimes up to six weeks. If your aerobic class is at fault, find a less stressful exercise until you heal. Swimming or bike riding are good alternatives," according to Dr. Griffin.

Side Stitches. "If you develop a stitch, stop running," advise Mona Shangold, M.D., and Gabe Mirkin, M.D., authors of *The Complete Sports Medicine Book for Women.* "Push your fingers deep into your belly just below your ribs on the right side. At the same time, purse your lips tightly and blow out as hard as you can. This should release the pressure on your diaphragm and stop the stitch—and you can be off and running again, pain free!"

Wracked Testicles. "Draw your legs up in a lying or sitting position to relieve the agony, and wait it out," Dr. Griffin advises. "It will seem endless, but the pain usually lasts just a couple of minutes. If the pain remains acute, see a doctor. If there's a nagging pain longer than a week, see a doctor. Use acetaminophen over aspirin here to cut down on the chance of internal bleeding. Don't use topical pain relievers and avoid soaks for the first day. After a day, a warm water soak in a bathtub or pool can help.

"If you have increased swelling or the pain goes to the stomach, you may have testicular torsion. See a doctor immediately," he says.

Chafed Nipples. "Joggers generally have this problem. The solution is to grease up the nipples. Petroleum jelly covered by a bandage or moleskin helps," says Dr. Griffin. "Wearing a soft cotton or silk jersey will keep

the pain from increasing. If the nipples become infected, see a doctor."

Breaks. "To test how bad the break is, press the fingernail or toenail of the affected limb. It should turn white, then pink. If it stays white, don't move the person at all. Call a paramedic and get an ambulance," Dr. Griffin instructs.

"In the meantime, keep the limb comfortable and immobile to avoid excess pain. Use anything stiff as a splint, but don't force the arm or leg into a position. Loosely apply it. An air splint is a nice thing to have around. You just sleeve the area and pump it up," he says.

Sports Burns. Falling, sliding, skidding, tackling, pinning—they're all a big part of sports. They can also give you one of the most painful forms of minor sports injuries—a friction burn.

"Grass, turf and mat burns are usually superficial, but they can give you the damndest infection you'll see in your life," says Dr. Richard Knutson. "That's because there's a lot of dirt and bacteria involved. You treat sports burns in one simple way— wash, wash, wash, a minimum of 10 to 15 minutes, using soap and water. It's going to hurt, but you've got to wash it off or it will hurt more later."

Injured Eyes. "If you injure your eyeball in any way, you must see an ophthalmologist," insists Dr. Arthur N. Landau. "The pain can be terribly severe, and ice won't help. In fact, there's a danger in any attempt to relieve the pain. You can take codeine or other oral painkillers, but that can fool you into thinking the injury is less serious because the pain has subsided. This may prevent you from going to the hospital for the treatment you need to save your sight.

"If you want to avoid this severe pain, you should wear eyeguards, especially when playing racquetball," he advises. "And you must wear the closed ones made from polycarbonate. There are no open eyeguards that are safe because a hard-hit ball can conform to the size of the opening and injure the eye to the same extent as if you were not wearing any protection at all."

Bob Kuechenberg
Miami, Fla.
Sports Injuries

"I've had my share of pain."

That comment—muttered by 6-time National Football League All-Pro offensive guard Bob Kuechenberg—should arch some eyebrows at the *Guinness Book of World Records*. It surely ranks as one of the all-time great understatements. Consider the scars of Big Bob's 15-year career with the 2-time Super Bowl champion Miami Dolphins.

"I've had a pair of broken toes, my right foot broken, torn ligaments in the arch and both ankles shattered, torn ligaments in my right knee, broken ribs, a broken back and a separated shoulder. I've had disk problems in the neck, two concussions, a broken left arm and numerous broken fingers. I broke my nose six times."

Despite this, Bob rarely missed a game. His record of starting 197 games (4 Super Bowls) ranks near the top for his position. He once played a full game with a broken ankle, and played the entire 1977 season with a broken back.

What is his secret? A fierce mental tenacity that overpowers the gnawing pain in his body.

"More than anything else, it was a matter of purpose. I was determined to recover from my injuries and keep playing football. My essence is as a football player.

"I would use ice after the injuries, and I applied heat to warm up prior to working out. Aside from that, where I may have had the edge is I was always well prepared physically and mentally. I paid a lot of attention to proper diet and supervised training. I took protein supplements in powdered form and a lot of vitamins—healthy doses of C, B complex and E.

"I also maintained an ironclad personal philosophy. I was never real big or real fast (a mere 6'2", 255), but my philosophy was, 'You may be able to beat me, but you'll have to kill me to do it.' I had the same attitude about pain. After I was injured, I exercised hard to get back in shape."

Hubert Rosomoff, M.D., a neurosurgeon at the University of Miami who specializes in pain, says such mental will power can actually block pain.

"If you exercise hard, you can overload the system by producing so much pain you blow the fuse on the pain relays and the pain disappears. Your body produces its own stress-induced analgesia," Dr. Rosomoff explains.

"It was all mental," Bob adds. "You play hurt, that's all."

7

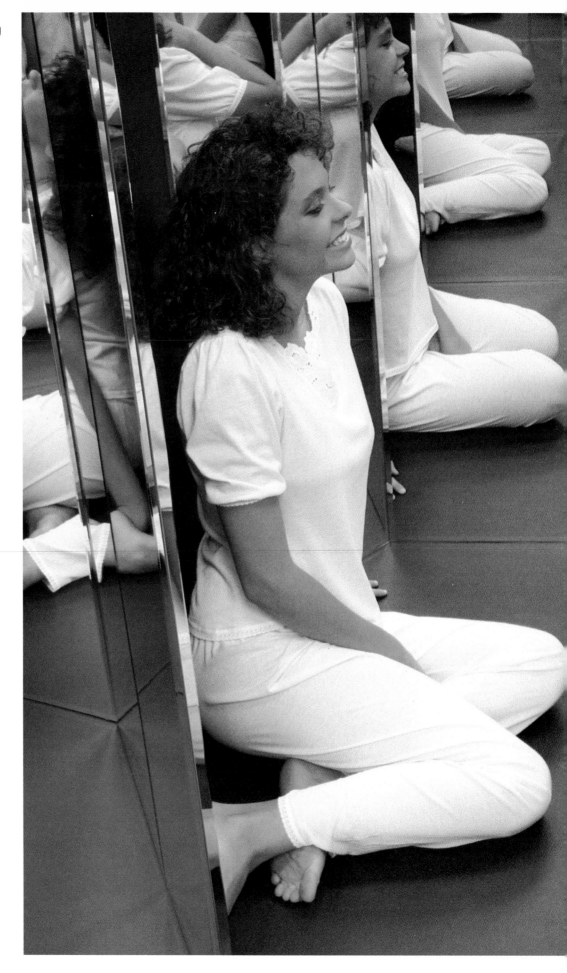

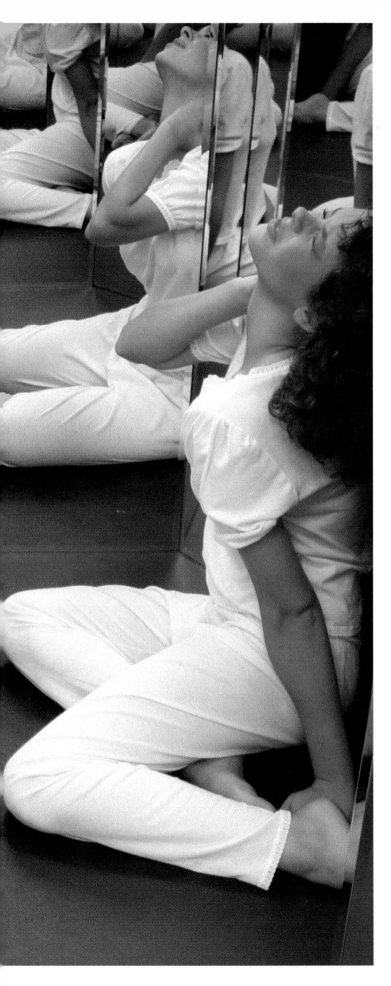

Changing the Painful Personality

Pain that won't go away doesn't have to be a life sentence. Discover how to break free.

"**Y**ou've had a toothache, haven't you? Well, imagine the worst toothache you've ever had. Now imagine that all the dentists in the world have died."

That, explains a man with nonstop spasms of the lower back, is how chronic, constant pain can make you feel—alone, hopeless, helpless. For Joseph, it began when he heard the cable snap before his elevator car plunged 35 feet to a sudden and painful stop. For Mary, it was when a mechanical, moving dance floor malfunctioned and crushed her leg. For Cy, it started when he fell down a steel ladder onto his spine.

At first they all looked forward to complete recovery and an end to their pain. But that end never came. "The injury has healed," the doctors said. "The pain should be gone." But time passed and the pain remained. Worry gave way to despair.

Some doctors offered them painkillers that only added to their problems. Others told them, "It's all in your head. You're crazy. You're doing it for attention, to get sympathy, to get money. You're lazy. You're faking."

The truth is, they were in pain. Real pain that became a constant companion that ruled their lives, breeding fear, hostility, anger, depression— and more pain. Suspicious insurance companies, insensitive friends and lack of a job added to the pressure.

And they weren't the only ones affected. Families can be torn apart at the seams by confusion and despair when a member gives in to the fear and depression that always follow chronic pain. Tempers flare. Harsh words replace kind thoughts.

But they—and thousands of others like them—have found ways to cheat pain of its psychological victory and to regain control of their lives. How? An accurate medical diagnosis of the

Hope Is Best

"The miserable," Shakespeare wrote, "have no other medicine but only hope."

What Shakespeare didn't know is that hope *is* a medicine. Shlomo Breznitz, Ph.D., an Israeli scientist, says when a person "practices" hope, the body may manufacture brain chemicals called endorphins that actually cut pain levels. Proof is supplied in part by a study of Israeli soldiers. The levels of hormones that indicate stress and anxiety were lowest in those soldiers who knew just how many miles were left in a long march. Knowing how far they had to go gave them hope, say the researchers, triggering a positive thought pattern that made the pain and fatigue easier to bear.

problem. Family therapy. Training for a new career. Laughing. Getting together with others in pain and letting them help. Learning relaxation techniques that help when the pain and stress are at their worst.

These solutions apply to all types of chronic pain, severe and mild, explains clinical psychologist Sheldon Levin, Ph.D., of the Mensana Clinic in Stevenson, Maryland. "You don't need the dramatics of having fallen down an elevator shaft to have constant pain," he says. "Or to learn how to live a rich, full life despite that pain."

Changing your attitude is the key to changing your life. As Aristotle once noted, "Happiness depends upon ourselves."

THE FOUR STAGES OF CHRONIC PAIN

Those facing the challenge of living with chronic pain go through four stages.

Stage One. "During the first stage, a person in chronic pain fully expects to get well," explains Dr. Nelson Hendler of Johns Hopkins. "They aren't depressed, even if the pain is severe."

Stage Two. "After the pain lasts more than two months, fear comes into play. We've always been told that pain means something is physically wrong," explains Dr. Hendler, who also runs the Mensana Clinic. "So there is anxiety and concern over the body.

"But," assures Dr. Hendler, "it's absolutely normal for a perfectly well-adjusted individual to become anxious and fearful when normal healing doesn't occur."

Stage Three. After they've been in pain for six months or longer, people reach what Dr. Hendler calls the chronic stage. That's when they begin to get very depressed. They've been to a lot of doctors and now worry that they'll have this pain for the rest of their life.

"This is when you have to convey to that person that there *is* a light at the end of the tunnel. Depressions *do*

get better. The psychological problems that accompany chronic pain will get better even though the pain may remain the same," says the doctor.

Stage Four. "They're going to feel better and function better because they'll be less depressed as they approach the fourth stage when they become more accepting of their condition," he says.

But acceptance doesn't mean false hope. "It's inappropriate to tell someone that one day they'll wake up and their pain will be gone. The real hope you can give them is that things are going to get better—that their level of functioning will improve.

"Very often a person in pain will say that the pain controls their life," explains Dr. Hendler. "It's important—for you as a pain patient—to understand that you can gain some temporary control over the pain. There are tools you can use to combat that feeling of helplessness, to have some control over your own environment.

"In some cases, the fight itself can be medically and psychologically therapeutic, depending on the kind of pain we're talking about," he says.

Diagnosing the cause of the pain is round one in that fight, says Dr. Hendler, because when you know exactly what you are up against, you are better able to do battle. At the Mensana Clinic, he insists on a specific medical diagnosis for each patient. "You say chronic pain to me," he explains, "and I think of 475 possible diagnoses."

But psychosomatic pain isn't one of them. Dr. Hendler has had too many patients referred to his clinic with a diagnosis of "psychogenic pain," "pain neurosis" or "malingering" who actually were suffering from entirely physical conditions like herniated disks, osteomyelitis (a bone disease) or reflex sympathetic dystrophy (a nervous system disorder).

"These are people whose pain had been labeled imaginary, yet they had a real problem that was going untreated because it hadn't been diagnosed yet." Even worse, continues Dr. Hendler, "some of these patients had become so brainwashed from hearing that their pain wasn't real that they had begun to doubt it themselves!

"One of the most important things you can tell someone in chronic pain is, 'If your doctor tells you the pain is in your head, get out of his office and find yourself another doctor.'"

Dr. Hendler's search for a correct diagnosis has uncovered a hidden medical problem in more than 20 percent of the patients who were referred to him with "imaginary" pain. For many, identifying the real cause of pain leads to a course of treatment that may cure or at least help reduce the level of pain.

HOW MUCH DO YOU HURT?

For others, a correct diagnosis leads to learning one of the many pain control techniques taught today. In these cases, the first step is a deceptively simple one: determining the level of pain. Yet pain is almost impossible to quantify. No doctor can see it and no medical machine or laboratory test can measure it. Then how can you measure it?

One way that you can measure actual pain intensity is by drawing a line about 4 inches long. One end represents no pain, while the other end means the worst pain imaginable. You then mark the point on the line that best represents your pain, and use a ruler to give it a number. Daily use of this "visual analogue" will show the ups and downs of the pain quite accurately, says Ronald Melzack, Ph.D., research director of Montreal General Hospital's pain center.

But it only measures intensity. Pain can be characterized by a variety of different sensations. Some pains burn; others stab; some cramp or sting. While some specialists recommend that you *not* talk about your pain or that you try and find "nicer" words to describe it, Dr. Melzack disagrees. He feels that accurately defining the various qualities of the pain, "frequently provides the key to diagnosis and may even suggest the best type of therapy."

The McGill-Melzack pain questionnaire was developed to give people a vocabulary to help them accurately describe their pains. The words it offers (see "Measuring Your Pain") were put together over a period

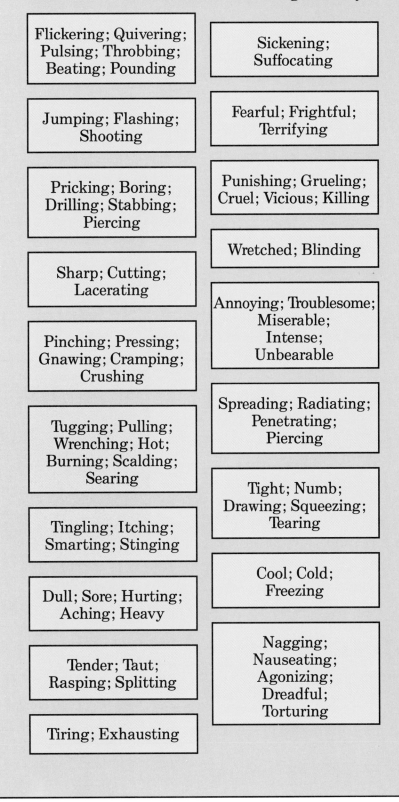

Measuring Your Pain

Pain can be hard to explain. Each of the boxes below offers you word choices that describe the intensity of different painful sensations. Use these words in your journal to help yourself see improvement as the pain is being treated. The words in each box are listed in order of increasing intensity.

Flickering; Quivering; Pulsing; Throbbing; Beating; Pounding

Jumping; Flashing; Shooting

Pricking; Boring; Drilling; Stabbing; Piercing

Sharp; Cutting; Lacerating

Pinching; Pressing; Gnawing; Cramping; Crushing

Tugging; Pulling; Wrenching; Hot; Burning; Scalding; Searing

Tingling; Itching; Smarting; Stinging

Dull; Sore; Hurting; Aching; Heavy

Tender; Taut; Rasping; Splitting

Tiring; Exhausting

Sickening; Suffocating

Fearful; Frightful; Terrifying

Punishing; Grueling; Cruel; Vicious; Killing

Wretched; Blinding

Annoying; Troublesome; Miserable; Intense; Unbearable

Spreading; Radiating; Penetrating; Piercing

Tight; Numb; Drawing; Squeezing; Tearing

Cool; Cold; Freezing

Nagging; Nauseating; Agonizing; Dreadful; Torturing

of almost 40 years and include suggestions from doctors, nurses and people in pain.

It was created so that health professionals could judge whether treatments were actually affecting the pain. But it led to the discovery that you could often diagnose the cause of a person's problem just by using the words they picked from the list. Each painful condition, it seems, has its own distinctive set of descriptive words.

"Once you've established that diagnosis," says Dr. Hendler, "you can begin to set some realistic goals. Most important, you can tell just how much a person can do physically without causing any further damage. A critical concept in eliminating some of the fear is that people can have pain and still function—still do things—without doing additional damage. They won't end up a cripple.

"But first you've got to make that diagnosis," stresses Dr. Hendler. "It opens up the whole rest of the world. It tells you prognosis, it tells you treatment, it tells you the appropriate course of counseling."

KEEPING TRACK OF YOUR PAIN

Keeping a journal, or pain diary, can provide you with valuable clues for making a diagnosis, as well as help you see patterns in your pain over a period of time.

Careful analysis of the entries can also reveal "what kind of situations in your life specifically give rise to painful symptoms" so that you can avoid them in the future, says Emmett E. Miller, M.D., a California physician who has created a series of relaxation and guided imagery tapes to ease many kinds of pain (see "Pain Relief in a Cassette" on page 102).

"Chronic pain is not constant," explains Dr. Miller. "It comes and goes. But people in pain don't notice that. Just as people with insomnia actually sleep several hours longer than they report, people in chronic pain forget that their pain levels rise and fall.

"The idea of a diary is to remind you that sometimes it's better and sometimes it's worse," he explains. Reading back over your diary teaches

you exactly what type of behavior precedes a painful episode. "That can help you change the behavior that produces the tension that gives rise to your chronic pain."

There are two parts to such a journal, explains David E. Bresler, Ph.D., psychologist and author of *Free Yourself from Pain*. In the first part, you simply rate your pain daily on a scale from 1 to 10.

When you look back at these ratings after several weeks, explains Dr. Bresler, you may be able to spot patterns that you didn't know existed. What were you doing when the pain was high on the scale? When it was low? Part two holds the answers.

That's the section Dr. Bresler calls the life chart. Just like a diary, it should include notations on:

- Your noteworthy experiences.
- Significant conversations.
- What you're thinking.
- Your emotional status.
- Any recent dreams.
- Your instinctive feelings.
- Any changes in your life.
- Plans for the future.
- Anything else you wish.

"Only if you are honest and thorough in your entries," emphasizes Dr. Bresler, "will you be able to see how your life progresses over an extended period of time." He suggests that you keep entries short, make them as soon as possible after an experience occurs and be sure to write *something* down at least once a day.

DO IT YOUR WAY

But don't worry about the format. Even though Betty Jane Gregor's pain journals (see "A Page from a Pain Journal") follow no strict guidelines, they overflow with useful information about the progression of her disease, physical events in her life and how she was feeling at the time.

"The writing itself is therapeutic," she says, "and the information may be helpful in charting the progress of the disease." (Also see Betty Jane's case history on page 41.)

Phil Dunphy, a physical therapist, agrees. "Pain patients are really playing

A Page from a Pain Journal

17 Oct: Dr. B. released me from the hospital. Said I have acute rheumatoid arthritis which is active. When I first entered the hospital my left wrist was badly swollen and the pain so great that it created symptoms of ulcers or gall bladder – nausea so bad I lost 10 pounds in 3 days time.

25 Nov: About 2 weeks after leaving the hospital, the pain started in my right shoulder. Several days later in the three small toes of my left foot. Just this morning, for the first time, pain in my jaw on the right side when I open my mouth. Using the paraffin baths once or twice a day for thirty minutes.

28 Nov: The pain in my left wrist seems to be moving out towards the fingers. Swelling is down to what I suppose will be normal for me for the rest of my life. My right shoulder seems to have more motion. I keep it moving as much as possible.

5 Dec: I have been sleeping with a wool sock on my left wrist and also on my left foot. There seems to be less pain and more movement in the morning since starting this. Food seems to have no taste since my jaw started to hurt.

26 Dec: The pain has lessened to such a degree that it seems as if it will go away altogether. Swelling in my left wrist has gone down even more. Still using paraffin. Knees only bother me occasionally. Left foot is more swollen than the right one. My shoulder is sore in the way a muscle becomes tender when unaccustomed to exercise. It bothers me a great deal at night. I am still one stiff 'board' in the morning, but all-in-all I am quite proud of my progress.

detective when they take notes on themselves," explains the director of H.E.A.R. (Health through Exercise and Rehabilitation), a fitness facility in Red Bank, New Jersey, where pain patients often develop a better attitude as a result of working out (see chapter 8).

"The only way a person in pain can learn the limits of what they can and can't do," explains Dunphy, "is by keeping track of when it hurts and how much it hurts."

SEXUAL SUCCESS

Sometimes that hurting can be a barrier to a healthy love life. When this problem occurs, Dunphy and his staff "spend a lot of time with the person explaining different positions they can use to have sex."

Most people in pain like the idea that sex can lessen pain for a time (see "Sextra-Strength Pain Relief" on page 96), but are frank in admitting that maintaining a normal sex life can be difficult.

"Freud pointed out that if there are any emotional difficulties, they're probably going to be expressed in the bedroom," explains Dr. Levin. "And people who've been in pain for awhile are going to become irritable, depressed, anxious, frustrated and hostile."

Dr. Levin has found that a

Betty Jane Gregor, whose arthritis case history appears on page 41, has kept journals detailing the progression of her arthritis and the events in her life for more than 20 years. It's a record of good days and bad ones, of advances and setbacks. In 1964 she wrote that "This epistle was started because it has just occurred to me that sometime some doctor may want to know or I may try to recall how this all started—and continued."

combination of both psychological and physical counseling "can help these people to still have pleasure, even with physical difficulties due to the pain. And that's very important. There's a give and take of feelings between two people that *needs* to be preserved."

And, says Dr. Levin, "there *are* people out there with tremendous pain who refuse to let it interrupt their sex lives or disrupt their families. They're the ones who are willing to relearn how to live their lives, who can accept a different way of doing things."

PAIN: ALL IN THE FAMILY

Since people in chronic pain tend to become estranged from everyone around them—not just their bed partners—the pain soon becomes a problem for the entire family. Nate, a member of a support group for people with chronic pain, explains:

"When I fell apart, the whole family fell apart," he remembers. "I could see it happening. I'd hear myself screaming at my wife and kids for talking too loud, but they weren't really loud—it was just the pain that made it seem that way."

"Even without a member in chronic pain, a family is always struggling to keep its balance," says Dr. Levin. "Pain can tip it over.

"But if the patient is supported by his family and if that support continues, they'll all survive the experience," he adds. To do that, "the kids need to understand that Daddy's in pain even though he may look fine, that he can't play with them as much even though he may be around the house more.

"But they can't reinforce *negative* behavior," he warns. "The family has to be careful not to make the patient feel like he can't function, that he shouldn't *try* to do things. They have to let him go at his own pace, while still trying to get him to function more.

"It's important for the family to avoid guilt trips—not to say, 'Well, you just don't want to take us anywhere.' That's why family therapy is extremely important. It can help define the medical limitations of what the person in pain can and can't do, so that the rest of the family knows what they can expect. Almost anyone can sit down at the table and do a jigsaw puzzle with their family, for instance," Dr. Levin concludes.

These are lessons that Nate had to learn. "I was grouchy all the time," he admits, because he couldn't take the family hunting like he had before he was crushed against the steering wheel of his truck. "Now I take them fishing, even if all I can do is bait the hook."

But, Nate admits, there are some aspects of his life that haven't been as easy to restore. "Sometimes I'll look at my wife and the tears just come to my eyes. This has aged her so much.

"The pain took away the glow we had for each other," he says, his eyes expressing his feelings as much as his words. "I realize now that what I have to do is pick up and start from day one to try and bring that glow back."

But Nate's task is easier because he has the help of others in pain.

Sextra-Strength Pain Relief

Sex as a pain reliever?

"I can tell you that it gets rid of a headache," offers one medical professional, "but that's just from personal experience."

Researchers at Rutgers came to the same conclusion in a controlled study. They found that women who were experiencing sexual pleasure could tolerate between 40 and 75 percent more pain than they could otherwise. The researchers also noted that the sex acted as a true analgesic—a pain *reliever*—rather than as an anesthetic that deadens all sensations.

More proof came from arthritis patients who were being studied at Cook County Hospital in Chicago. Wanda Sadoughi, M.D., explains that the patients reported that they were completely free of pain for several hours after having sex.

Robert, Linda and Wade Wilson Aberdeen, Md. Chronic Pain

One night, Linda Wilson heard noises coming from their 2-year-old son's room. Wade was talking in his sleep. "Daddy," she heard him say, "I'm just a little baby, don't get mad at me!" Watching her son toss and turn, she realized that pain was destroying her family.

Wade was 8 months old when she took him along to pick up her husband after work. They passed a man covered with blood, sitting by the side of the road. Something clicked and she turned the car around. The hat and T-shirt were unmistakable. That was her *husband* under all that blood.

A heavy equipment operator, Robert had stepped out from under his machine's protective canopy and been struck on the head by a tree limb that had fallen 75 feet. The impact knocked him off the platform and down to the ground, onto his head.

His skull was fractured in 10 places. An operation put his face back together, but nothing could stop the pain. "I'd just be walking down the street," he says, "and ZAP!—it'd feel like someone hit me in the head with a baseball bat."

Red tape delayed his compensation checks as well as essential medical treatments. He became, he says, "like a stick of dynamite with a short fuse."

Arguments would spark the explosion. When the pressures got to Linda, she'd remind him that *she* was the only one working. "Then I'd get mad and say a lot of things I'd regret later," admits Robert.

Just as Linda was ready to leave him, Robert entered a clinic for a month-long stay.

Two weeks later came a revelation. "I was up late with some of the patients from my group therapy," he recalls. "I was feeling bad about the problems they were having at home when I realized— Hey! That sounds like me! I'm in the same boat, doing the same things to my wife."

The next time Linda came to visit, Robert was waiting with flowers he had picked from the grounds. "I think the last time I had given her flowers was while we were dating, about 13 years before." He apologized for "being ignorant," and said that he wanted to change.

"The counselors at the clinic helped Robert to see that he was demanding perfection from his family because he couldn't get it from himself anymore," explains Linda. "He had been jumping on Wade—a 2-year-old—like he was an adult."

"I had turned my house into a battlefield," says Robert. "When we had a fight, I'd *stay* mad. Now they last 5 minutes and we make up. It was the pain. The pain made me irritable, unreasoning. My thinking wasn't right at all. It made me evil."

The clinic helped reduce some of that pain. But most important, says Robert, "it helped me get rid of my 'stinking thinking.'"

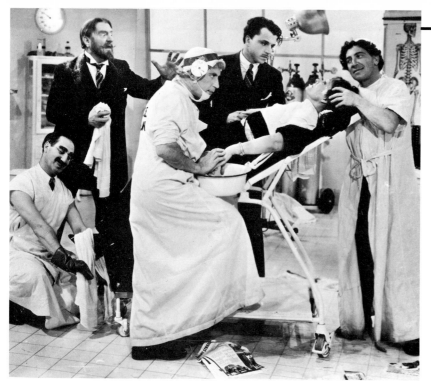

They say you should laugh till it hurts—but what in the world could ever seem funny to someone in serious pain? Comedienne Carol Burnett came up with a routine *about* pain that should make just about anyone laugh. Since men can't actually experience childbirth, she wanted to give them some idea of what labor pains feel like: "Take your bottom lip," she said, "and pull it over your head." That's a good line. And a good line can bring good health. E. Forrest Boyd, M.D., wrote that laughter aids the circulation, massages the abdominal muscles, stimulates digestion, lowers blood pressure, "begets optimism and self-confidence and relegates fear and pessimism to the background." Pain just can't survive a good laugh. If there were a single drug that could accomplish the same, it'd be worth—or cost—a million bucks. So have a cheap laugh instead.

YOU ARE NOT ALONE

"The worst part of chronic pain is the feeling of being hopeless and helpless," explains Mary E. Davidson, a licensed clinical social worker, who organizes support groups for the Mensana Clinic. "Feeling that you *can* do something is real important." And the people best qualified to get that message across are others in pain.

"Nobody in the outside world really understands chronic pain," explains one member of the group. "And so I didn't want to be around those other people because I wasn't like they were anymore. I was uneasy with everybody.

"But just coming here and talking to others that were like me—and some that were worse off—and hearing their point of view helped me a lot. I realized that I wasn't the only one going through this, and if the others could learn to accept it, *I* had to learn to accept it.

"It's been five or six years and it's *still* hard sometimes. But whenever something goes wrong and I start to get emotional, I think of everyone here and say to myself, 'why am I acting this way when there are others who are even worse?'"

Another member agrees. "The main thing about the group," she feels, "is that you're with people who understand your pain and what it's doing to you. I can talk about things here that I still can't discuss with my family.

"It's just like in Alcoholics Anonymous," she continues. "The people here have been where you're at, and they can help you over the rough spots. When someone new comes into the group we share our experiences with them, and let them know what *we* did to get ourselves through those hard times."

There are other benefits as well. "One of the people in the group brought up that he was having trouble remembering things, and the others all said that they were having that problem, too," she recounts. The culprit, they discovered, was the pain, not some mental deficiency.

"We'd channel all our energy into trying to reduce and deal with the pain," says one veteran member about the problem, "and our minds just wouldn't function as well because we were taking so much of that energy away from them."

Assurances from other members that they were all having the problem served to reduce the fear that something terrible was happening. "It made us realize we weren't getting senile."

Sometimes that reassurance is all that's needed to eliminate the memory problem. Ms. Davidson notes that "people's concentration usually improves once they've been reassured that this is part of the normal process of pain."

Dr. Levin sees yet another benefit. "Group therapy gives a person in pain the opportunity to help others," he explains. "That new perspective as helper allows them to look at themselves in a new light. If they can help others, they can certainly regain some control over their own lives."

But the main benefit of being in a group, he feels, is "having to look at all these *other* people with tough breaks. You can't stay isolated in that kind of a situation. You have to come out of your shell and get on with your life. And learning to live a productive life actually makes the pain less because you're not sitting around dwelling on it."

In fact, you may even be laughing at it.

I ONLY LAUGH WHEN I HURT

"We can laugh at one another in here in spite of all our pain," explains an older group member.

Many of the members will explain, while wiping tears of laughter out of their eyes, that they hadn't laughed for years before joining the group. "Now they'll laugh and joke their way through an entire 1½-hour session," says Ms. Davidson. "It's a tremendous release for them."

Dr. Levin feels that regaining that ability to laugh at yourself and your pain—even when the subject is as somber as going without sex or the inability to clean yourself in the bathroom—is an important step. "There's that understanding that you *can* change your perspective and have a better attitude.

"Before you can escape the pain," he explains, "you have to stop thinking of yourself as a martyr. You have to stop being morose."

Morose is something that other members of the group will not let you be. "Sometimes I feel like I'm running a bar without liquor," says Dr. Hendler of the days that a support group meets at his clinic. "This is their gathering spot."

HAPPY HEALING

Laughing may provide more than just a way to a better attitude. Much evidence suggests that good humor may be good pain medicine.

William McDougall, Ph.D., former professor of psychology at Harvard University, wrote in 1922 that laughter is "primarily and fundamentally an antidote of . . . pain," that works in two ways. "First, laughter interrupts the train of mental activity; it diverts or rather relaxes the attention.

"Secondly, the bodily movements of laughter hasten the circulation and respiration and raise the blood pressure, and so bring about a condition of euphoria or general well-being which gives a pleasurable tone to consciousness."

Raymond A. Moody, M.D., who explored "the healing power of humor" in his book, *Laugh after Laugh,*

proposes that "having a good sense of humor" really means the ability "to acquire a cosmic perspective on one's problems."

Ms. Davidson looks at it another way. "Laughter is like sex," she says. "It's hard to feel the pain when you're in the middle of it."

THE PAIN OF UNEMPLOYMENT

But it's hard to enjoy either of those desirable distractions when your pain is so bad you can't work—and you want to. In fact, your pain is probably *worse* if you're unemployed. Subjects of a study presented at a meeting of the American Public Health Association were more "concerned with bodily symptoms than those who continued to work."

That's why Dr. Hendler urges his patients to get vocational counseling while battling their pain problems. This type of counseling has to deal with unique problems.

That's because the road to employment can be an obstacle course of barriers and pitfalls, especially for those who were injured on the job. All too frequently, old employers hold your injury against you or offer a lower position at less pay. A new employer may be reluctant to pay for your medical insurance or may have a real fear that you'll reinjure yourself—at the company's expense.

Even worse, some pain patients find themselves hounded by their previous employer, or the employer's insurance company. Take the case of a middle-aged man with a serious back injury incurred on the job. He was encouraged by his doctor to try to do more physical things around the house. It might hurt, the doctor explained, but the activity wouldn't cause any further damage.

But when the man went outside to bring in some firewood, his wife spotted a man hiding in the trees spying through a camera with a telescopic lens. It was a private detective hoping to get pictures of the man doing things around the house so that the insurance company could dispute his claim.

A case like this could lead the insurance company to say in court: "You're not hurt. We saw you out

Employment and Pain

Chronic pain is enough of a problem at home, but how do you present this problem when you're applying for a job? And what can you do if the pain starts to interfere with your work after you're hired?

"If you can cope with your pain and the requirements of the job don't make it worse, it shouldn't be an issue when you apply for the job," explains Paul G. Hearne. He's the executive director of Just One Break, Inc., in New York City, the oldest job placement service for the disabled in the nation.

For pain to be a problem, he explains, "it must affect the particular functions of the job you are applying for or currently hold. It's just like any other disability—unless the pain affects your ability to do the job, it's not relevant."

When you look for a job, having reasonable goals is the key to avoiding future disappointment, says Hearne. There's a much greater chance of long-term success if you define and seek out jobs that make use of your best skills and aren't unduly interfered with by your pain.

If you get the job in good faith and find that your performance is limited by your pain, ask your employer to make reasonable accommodations to help you work. These are things like a stool to sit on, an electric typewriter instead of a manual, or a headset so you don't need to hold a phone all day.

If you have trouble working out an arrangement with your employer, contact your state's Vocational Rehabilitation office or the Rehabilitation Services Administration in Washington, D.C. They may suggest a program in your area, such as Projects with Industry, that can devise the correct procedures that will allow you to do your job and suggest easy ways for your boss to implement them.

And he probably will. It's been Hearne's experience that, "where you have a productive employee who wants to work and can do the job, the employer will work to keep them."

opposed to faking it for sympathy and money?

"The system," says Dr. Hendler, "is counterproductive to the care of the patient. Instead of everyone co-operating to get this guy back to work, the insurance company and workers' compensation board spend a lot of energy and money to try and 'catch' him cheating.

"Companies talk about the 'green poultice'—that's when your pain gets better as soon as the case is settled. But if you look at the figures carefully, even the workers who *do* win a settlement often wind up with much less than if they had been able to continue working," says Dr. Hendler.

GETTING BACK TO WORK

At many pain clinics, help in obtaining future employment comes in the form of a vocational guidance counselor, who puts the patient through a series of tests. The counselor then figures out the kinds of tasks that the patient can perform with the least pain, explains options and helps find the training that may lead to employment.

"Sensible placement and realistic goals" are the key to finding and keeping that new job, explains Paul G. Hearne, executive director of New York City's Just One Break, Inc., the oldest job placement service for the disabled in the nation. Hearne has achieved a remarkable 85 percent retention rate for his clients by carefully matching people with the right jobs. Sometimes that means giving up an unrealistic dream.

"We had an applicant with a degree in botany who also had a very painful knee trauma," explains Hearne. "He wanted desperately to apply for a park ranger's job that involved a lot of standing and required that he be able to perform CPR. We had to counsel him to look for another way to make use of that degree."

Sometimes, however, that new job can wind up better than the one left behind. "We had a fellow who worked as an electrician," recalls Dr. Hendler, "who was injured on the job. He went to rehab and learned computer repair. Now he has four people working for him and makes

lifting wood." Would the judge be enlightened enough to realize that the injured person is attempting to bravely struggle through his pain, as

triple what he did before he got hurt."

But more money doesn't mean less pain. Being employed, having soul sessions with like-minded friends, laughing—these can do only so much. At some point, you—by yourself—have to deal with the stress of chronic pain. And the best way to do that is to *relax*.

RELAXING AWAY THE PAIN

"When the probability of actual pain relief is small," says Dr. Levin, "the best thing you can do is to teach the patient relaxation exercises."

"It gives them another tool that they can use to combat that feeling of helplessness," continues Dr. Hendler. And he says that in some cases, such as migraine or tension headaches, "relaxation can be an actual therapy to get rid of the pain."

People in pain have a tendency to keep their muscles tensed all the time. Learning to relax those muscles may not affect the original pain problem directly, but it can take away any pain that is being "added on."

"Besides the primary pain," says Dr. Hendler, "these people have secondary pain from muscle tension and psychological stress. By reducing some of that secondary and psychological pain, you've helped the patient feel better."

There are many ways to relax. Some people do well listening to certain types of calming music (see "Sounds That Soothe" on page 103). Others prefer techniques such as biofeedback. And some respond well to prerecorded tapes that "guide" them through journeys of imagery, relaxation or behavior modification.

"But learning how to relax is not that easy," cautions Dr. Levin. "It's going to take a while. Once you learn to relax properly, however, it's like riding a bike or playing the piano. It's something you never forget."

Before you can learn to relax, you have to, well, relax. It's just not something you can force on yourself. "If you try too hard, it just won't work," warns Dr. Levin. And that makes sense. Think about someone with a really determined look on their face, muscles tensed, growling through gritted teeth: "Okay! Now

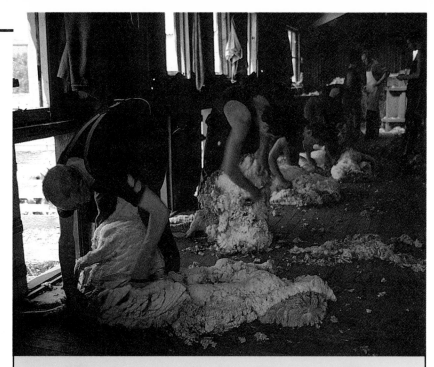

The System Makes Them Suffer

Researchers compared workers in New Zealand and the U.S. who were receiving disability payments for back pain and found that although pain among the two groups was about the same, the New Zealanders just didn't give in to it as much as the Americans. The reason: The U.S. compensation system *encourages* people to suffer.

The University of Virginia researchers say the Americans' lives were much more disrupted by the pain: They were more emotionally upset, used more medication and had more limited social, recreational and sex lives.

The New Zealanders, on the other hand, were quicker to resume their normal lives and get back to work. They needed less extra rest, and they didn't visit the doctor as often after their treatment program as the Americans.

Why? The researchers feel the compensation system in New Zealand contributes to less disability because—unlike the U.S. system—rehabilitation begins earlier, employers and insurance companies don't take an adversary position, and there are penalties for workers who refuse alternative employment.

I'm going to relax!"

Don't try to relax while the kids are roller skating inside the house or while the dog is leaping into your lap. Schedule some quiet time in a private room, with no distractions.

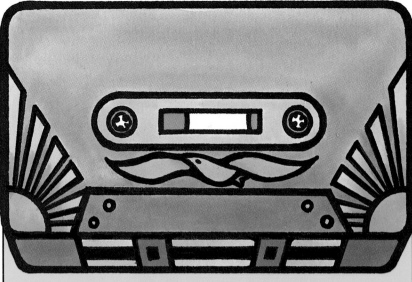

Pain Relief in a Cassette

Stuffed between the Cyndi Lauper and Michael Jackson cassettes at your local audio outlet are tapes that offer pain relief and relaxation instead of rock and roll. But how do you find the one that's right for you? Emmett E. Miller, M.D., author and narrator of the "Software for the Mind" series of tapes, has some suggestions. "Check with professionals—ask people at the local biofeedback clinic or someone who is doing relaxation therapy. Talk with your physician and see if it makes sense for you to listen to the tapes, and if they have any guidelines for you to follow.

"If *I* were the consumer, I would buy several different tapes on the same topic, listen to them all and see which one felt good to me. My belief is that when people listen, they can tell the quality difference between tapes: the basic enjoyability, or ease of listening; does the tape contain some wisdom, some truly effective techniques?

"You may wind up saving these tapes and using different ones to treat different pains. One may be just great at getting rid of your acute pain, while another may really help you to feel better about your long-term possibilities. I think that the tapes have so increased in their potential to improve people's lives over what was available, say, 10 years ago, that it would be silly not to buy them."

You can learn a relaxation technique from your therapist, listen to one of the many tapes that are available or try the following method.

TENSE UP TO RELAX

The Jacobsen method of relaxation is especially good if you're a beginner, since you can feel results quickly, and it diverts your mind from distractions such as worrying and thinking at 100 miles per hour. (Consult your doctor before using this technique because the movements can be counterproductive with some pains.)

As you practice this technique the first few times, pay special attention to those parts of your body that resist relaxation. Later on, you'll want to concentrate on these areas rather than going through the entire sequence.

As you get better at the technique, you might want to silently repeat a word like *relax* or *calm* in your mind every time you release the tension. With practice, that word or phrase alone may be enough to induce the feeling of relaxation. Here's how to do the Jacobsen method. Get comfortable. You can sit or lie down, whichever feels better. Close your eyes and let yourself relax. Attune yourself to your breathing. Don't control it, just listen to the air flow in and out through your nose.

After about a minute, you're going to begin tensing and then relaxing each part of your body. You'll want to hold each part tensed for about 6 seconds, then slowly let it relax and spend about 15 or 20 seconds just feeling the relaxation flow into that part of your body.

Ready?

Tense your right hand by making a fist. Hold it, then relax.

Tense and relax your right upper arm by bending it at the elbow and bringing your hand up to your shoulder.

Do the same for your left hand. Then your left upper arm.

Now your shoulders—lift them up toward your ears.

Tense your right foot and calf by bending the toes down toward the heel.

Now just your right calf—bend the big toe toward your knee.

The upper part of your right leg—lift it 6 inches off the ground.

Now do the same for your left

foot and calf, the calf alone and your left upper leg.

Tense and relax your neck by pushing your head back, then again by bringing your chin down toward your chest.

Tense and relax your forehead by frowning, then your eyes by squinting.

Do your lips by squeezing them together tightly, then your tongue by pushing it up against the roof of your mouth.

Clench your teeth together to tense the jaw.

Push your trunk upward to tense your chest.

Arch up for the back.

For your stomach, draw it in toward the backbone. Then reverse, pushing it outward.

After you've done all that once, go through the sequence again, but without tensing. Just savor the feeling of relaxation in each part and stay a little longer in the areas that still seem tense before moving on.

Then just sit or lie quietly. Enjoy that feeling of relaxation. Be calm and contented. It's okay to let your mind drift away, but don't let yourself start thinking about things. If you begin to concentrate on an issue, go back and focus on how your body feels.

Allow yourself 10 or 20 minutes for the entire experience, but don't watch the clock. Your eyes should still be closed as you slowly come back into the room by listening to the sounds around you. Slowly move your hands and feet a bit and then gradually open your eyes and allow them to get accustomed to the light. Get up very slowly and just savor the feeling for a bit.

Relaxing twice a day is best, but once is okay. If it seems difficult, don't give up—it should become easier with time. Distractions should slowly disappear with practice.

Don't perform the exercise until at least two hours after a meal. The best times are midmorning, midafternoon and shortly before supper.

"Stress relaxation is like working out," explains Ms. Davidson. "You do it a few times a week so that the strength is there when you need it. People shouldn't expect instant results—the relaxation response needs to be built up gradually."

Sounds That Soothe

What do classical guitar, Barbra Streisand's greatest hits, country and western music and the hard-core rock sounds of Alice Cooper have in common? They've all helped people reach the desired "alpha state" of consciousness during biofeedback training that reduces the extra stresses caused by chronic pain. *Familiar* music, it seems, is the key to achieving deeper relaxation.

Familiar *sounds* may work even better. Irv Teibel, president of Syntonic Research, Inc., in New York City, has captured sounds that he calls genetic experiences—thunderstorms, crashing surf, wind in the trees, even the human heart—on special records and cassettes designed for repeated playings. The sounds of nature contained in the "Environments" series of recordings calm the listener by transporting them to an ocean or a meadow where they can forget their pain for a bit.

Others, such as the "Software for the Mind" series of audio cassettes by Emmett E. Miller, M.D., combine music and environmental sounds with a relaxing voice. These tapes take listeners on "healing journeys" during which they learn how to ease physical pain—pain from chronic conditions and acute pains like pounding headaches.

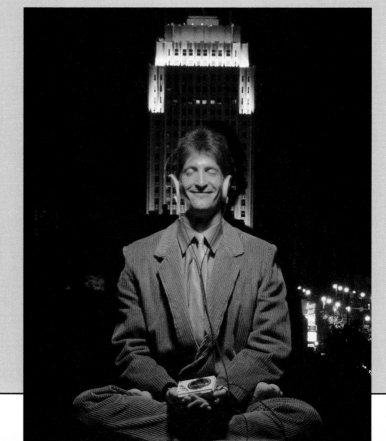

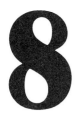

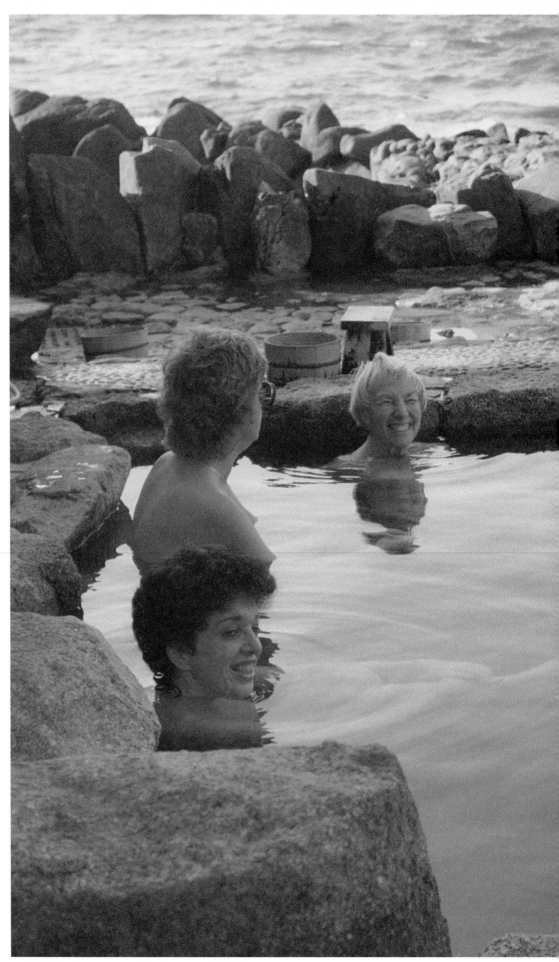

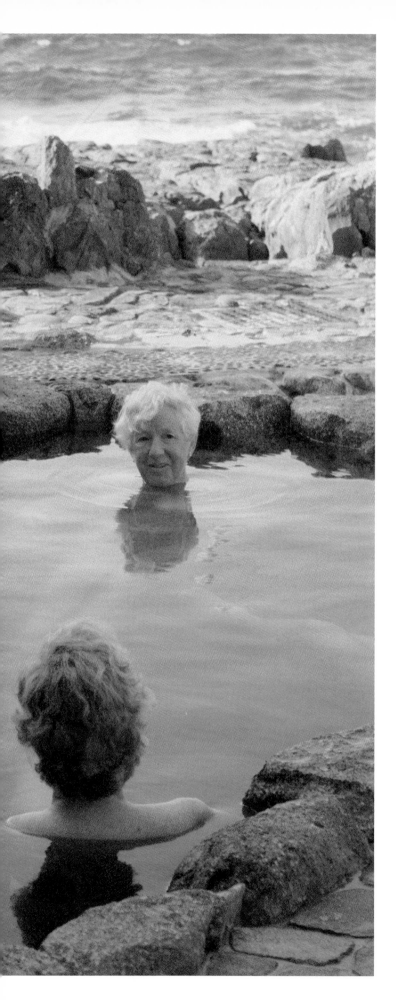

Hands-On Healing

A painful body loves the professional healing touch of the physical therapies.

Your body hurts. How *dare* it, you wail indignantly.

Didn't you slave all day, slumped at your desk or slinging 30-pound sacks around a construction site, just to keep *it* fed and sheltered? Didn't you keep going when *it* wanted to quit? But didn't you treat it to good things, too—like pizza, french fries and anything frosted and wrapped in cellophane?

And didn't you humor your body's desire for total sloth, most nights letting it collapse in a heap before the television set? You never demanded that it exercise—except, now and then, on weekends.

Where did you go wrong?

Everywhere.

"Of course it's hard not to feel betrayed when your body hurts," admits Alan Weiner, D.O., director of the pain control center at the Osteopathic Hospital of Maine in Portland. "But this attitude ignores *your* responsibility for the condition of your body."

You and your body are inseparable. Pain begins when upsets in your body are translated into "pain" by your mind. The upsets often result from a stressful life: too much work, too little exercise, poor diet. If your body were better taken care of, it would be less likely to ache.

This contention is shared by a wide variety of therapies, all of which emphasize direct manipulation of your body in the service of pain control. The therapies range from ice massage to supervised exercise. But all share one overriding concern: "We try, always, to allow the patient some measure of control over his own therapy and, by extension, over his own life," says Dr. Weiner.

In practice, this control can mean applying your own heating pad at home or religiously following the regimen recommended by your nutritionist. But, most important, it means learning to care for and work *with* your body. The two of you, together, are a powerful pain-fighting machine.

EVERYONE NEEDS TO BE KNEADED

If you're sore and sad, if your muscles ache, your head hurts, your

Homemade Massage Oil

There's really no need to purchase massage lotion at the store, because most brands are just mixtures that you can easily blend at home. Registered massage therapist Elliot Greene and his colleague Patricia Logan say to start with a base of any plant oil such as sweet almond, avocado, cocoa butter, coconut, olive, apricot, peanut or palm. (These aren't easily absorbed by your skin, and thus are better lubricants.) Then blend in an equal part of a more absorbable oil, such as soy or safflower. Add a few drops of perfumed oil—for example, musk, clove or frangipani— and you'll make a sensual experience even more so. Greene suggests you try this recipe:

Blend ⅓ cup each of peanut oil, cold-pressed soy oil and safflower oil. Add 3 or 4 drops of musk oil.

stomach churns and life in general is rubbing you the wrong way, try, for once, getting rubbed the *right* way: Try a massage.

"Massage is an effective way to deal with many kinds of pain," says Kerrith McKechnie, a registered massage therapist and director of the Potomac Myotherapy Institute in Washington, D.C. "It can't 'cure' illness or traumatic injuries. But for most people, it's a wonderful way to enhance total body health."

When someone mentions massage—especially professional massage—many of us chuckle, nudge one another and exchange knowing looks. But the massage that therapists practice and promote is not a form of sex. "Massage is a legitimate approach to pain relief, one that has both physiological and psychological benefits," stresses Ms. McKechnie. "And it's a great way to make yourself feel better."

What is massage's magic? How can it help you deal with, even dissipate, pain? First, it can help the pummeled muscle itself, answers Raymond J. Hruby, D.O., of San Diego, California.

Deeply massaging muscles helps reduce swelling in them, he explains. Since swelling is typically followed by stiffness, impaired motion and pain, massage—by deflating the swelling—helps relieve the pain.

Massage also increases blood flow to the muscles, says Dr. Hruby, hastening the removal of lactic acid and other by-products of muscle activity. These wastes can irritate nerve endings, causing sore muscles after exertion. Massage is especially beneficial if you're beginning or increasing an exercise regimen, because lactic acid buildup is greatest at these times.

But even if your pain has nothing to do with muscle by-products, massage can be valuable. Pain in general is often traceable to muscle spasms. These spasms are the body's way of immobilizing an ill or injured area. "The spasm is a protective action. It acts as a homemade splint, preventing movement in the affected part," Dr. Hruby says.

But this splint effect is counterproductive, because it causes extra pain and prevents the original illness

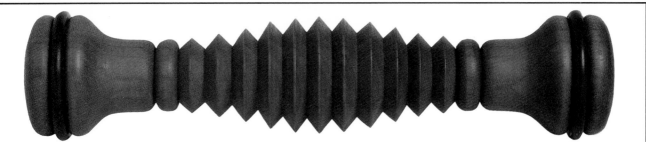

Home Massagers Can Rub You the Right Way

You've had a hard day—your feet are killing you, your head is pounding and your whole body is tense. Want a quick and easy way to relax? Try using one of the home massagers available at health, sporting goods and department stores. According to Boulder, Colorado, massage therapist Sharon Mason-Jordan, devices like body massagers, padded spinal rollers, shower massagers and wooden foot rollers (like the one shown above) can be quite effective if used properly.

While they aren't recommended for people with skeletal problems or recent injuries, at $10 to $40 the gadgets are an inexpensive way to treat muscle tension. But purchase them wisely. A friend's recommendation is good, says Ms. Mason-Jordan. Examine the quality of the material—wood is usually best. And check to see if detailed instructions are included.

As an alternative, you can save money by using equally effective household products. A rolling pin makes an excellent foot massager. Rolling your back over a small rubber ball loosens tight muscles, while padded paint rollers make fine substitutes for body massagers. Whatever the device, however, proper use is essential. Never use an unpadded roller directly on the spine, and don't apply too much pressure to any body area. Stop if you feel any pain, and don't massage an isolated area for more than 5 minutes at a time.

or injury from healing. Breaking up the spasm with massage not only alleviates the muscle pain, it also helps your body relax. In a relaxed, more healthful state you can better withstand the stress or injury that originally caused the pain.

Relaxation is only one of the psychological dividends of massage, though. "Massage helps you recognize your essential self-worth," says Ms. McKechnie. "You're being touched and cared for by someone, so you must be worthwhile. Just knowing this can give you the incentive to take better care of yourself, all the time."

THE BEST KINDS OF MASSAGE

If you're ready to rush out and get yourself professionally rubbed, stop for a minute and decide what kind of massage you want. Professional massage encompasses more than you might have imagined. "We don't believe in too narrow an interpretation of massage," Ms. McKechnie explains. "Purposeful touching of the body, with a therapeutic intent— that's a massage."

A definition this broad can encompass all the different kinds of massage. Western massage is probably the type you've been thinking of as massage. Popularized by a Swedish physiologist in the early 19th century (and thus often called Swedish massage), it involves a systematic stroking, kneading and pressing of the body's muscles, ligaments, tendons and skin. In addition to its direct effect on your tissue, Western massage takes aim against pain by inducing total relaxation.

Eastern massage, or shiatsu, is also used to relax you. But the methods and philosophy behind it are different. Although shiatsu has its origins in acupuncture, it doesn't involve needles. Instead the therapist will use finger pressure on various acupuncture points. The theory

(continued on page 110)

How to Give a Foot Massage

Try this age-old technique that really gets to the "sole" of your pain—foot massage. No matter what's hurting you, "for every important organ or muscle area in the trunk and head there is a tiny area that corresponds to it on one or both feet," says George Downing, author of *The Massage Book*. Massaging them may really give you an all-over, pain-relieving workout. What follows are Downing's directions for a great foot massage. He recommends little or no oil but considerable elbow grease—so press hard for best results.

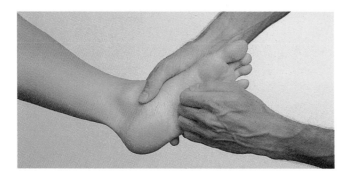

1 Choose a comfortable place to work. If you're using a massage table, have your partner lie on his or her back. Otherwise, seat your partner in a chair with one foot propped on a cushioned stool. Start by holding the top of the foot with one hand. Make a fist with the other and massage the entire sole with your knuckles, using tiny circular movements from heel to toe. Don't forget the bottom of the heel.

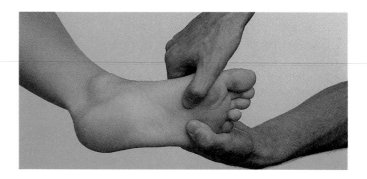

2 Now grasp the foot with both hands, thumbs on the sole. Massage the sole again with your fingers and thumbs, pressing in the same circular motions. Go very slowly and carefully—you don't want to miss any pain-relieving spots. And don't forget to use a lot of pressure (about the same force you'd use to push a thumbtack into a piece of wood).

3 Change your grip and vigorously massage the top of the foot from toes to ankle, using the same thumb motions. As you approach the ankle and heel, massage with your fingertips, but keep up the same circular pressure. Make sure to massage both the top and sides of the ankle, then end at the bottom of the heel.

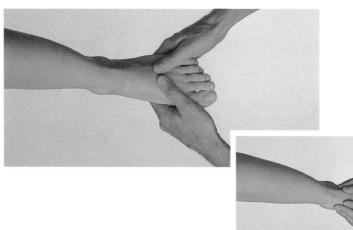

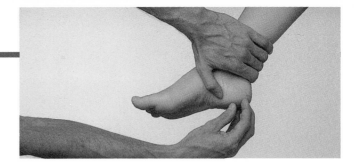

4 Once you reach the bottom of the heel, lift the foot from behind the ankle and use your fingertips and thumb of the opposite hand to slowly massage the bottom edge of the heel. Press firmly.

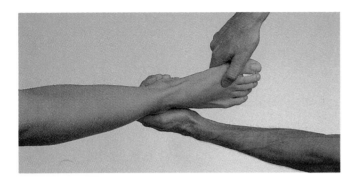

5 Now look at the top of the foot. See those long, thin tendons running from the ankle to the toes? Run the tip of your thumb down the valley between them, pressing hard. When you reach the flap of skin between the toes, give it a gentle squeeze before moving on to the next valley.

6 Now point your thumbs away from the toes and bring the heels of your hands together. Wrap your hands around the foot and press firmly in both directions—downward with the heels of your hands and upward with your fingertips against the middle of the sole. Continue steady pressure while slowly sliding the heels of your hands apart. When they reach the outer edges of the foot, start over. Do this 3 times.

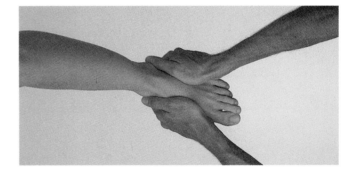

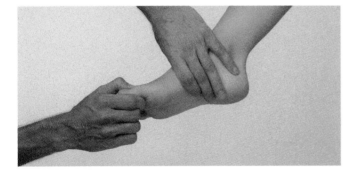

7 Hold the foot steady and massage the toes. Grasp the base of the big toe between your thumb and forefinger and pull gently. Twist it gently from side to side as if you were removing a cork from a bottle. Allow your fingers to slide off the tip. Do each toe in turn.

8 Finally, cool down the foot by clasping it between your palms, sandwich style. Hold it motionless for a few moments before moving on to the other foot.

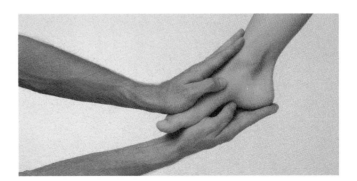

is that when these points are pressed, energy that is trapped within your body, producing pain or illness, is released.

Whichever type of massage therapist you choose, find one who is a member of the American Massage Therapy Association. These therapists have undergone rigorous train-ing. Some states also have licensing boards. Call your state's Division of Professional Licensing Services to find out if it can give you the names of licensed massage therapists in your area.

According to Ms. McKechnie, you can also practice massage easily and effectively on your own. "Buy a

Rinse Away Tension

Let your shower wash muscle stiffness and tension down the drain. Just aim the stream of warm water at the sore muscles and relax as you do these exercises devised by Lisa Dobloug, a Washington, D.C., fitness consultant. (Be sure to stand on a rubber mat to avoid slipping.)

Lower Back Release

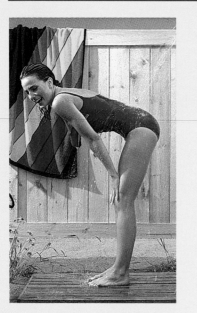

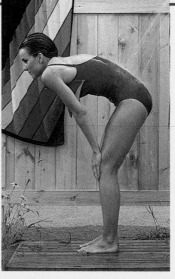

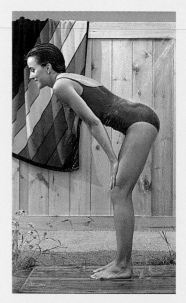

Stand with your feet hip width apart. Bend your knees slightly, hands rest-ing on your thighs, back straight, abdominals tightened.

Exhale, tuck in your tailbone and round your spine like an angry cat. Tighten your abdominal muscles and shift your pelvis forward. Feel the stretch through your lower back.

Reverse the sequence slowly and repeat 4 to 6 times.

book. Better yet, take a one-day seminar on massage techniques," she urges. "You and everyone you practice with will love it."

Perhaps even more important, you'll learn one of the most effective techniques for self-management of pain. "Massage requires that you tune into your body, to its problems and needs," Ms. McKechnie explains. "And isn't acting with, not against, your body the first step toward dealing with your body's pain?"

Absolutely, Dr. Hruby would say. As an osteopathic physician, he thinks the basic responsibility for pain control lies with you. He and other osteopaths view their role as

Total Back Stretch

Stand straight with your feet hip width apart. Exhale, slowly drop your head onto your chest, round your back and then bend at the hips, knees and ankles to lower your seat until your hands touch the floor. Let your arms, shoulders, neck and head hang. Feel the heaviness of your head. Inhale slowly and reverse the sequence, using your thighs and abdomen to raise you. Repeat 4 to 6 times.

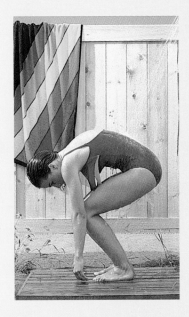

Side Stretch/Twist

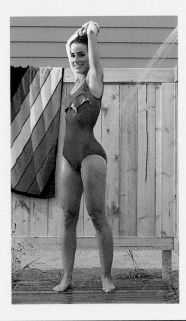

Stand tall, feet firmly planted. Clasp your forearms over your head, holding your shoulders down. Focus on your abdominal muscles. Inhale, then exhale, stretching to the right. Keep your waist still and your hips forward and centered. Inhale and return to the upright position. Repeat, stretching to the left. Then, standing tall with your hands on the opposite elbows, rotate your upper body to the right, keeping your hips facing forward. Then rotate left. Repeat the sequence 4 to 6 times. Inhale on rotation. Exhale on return to center.

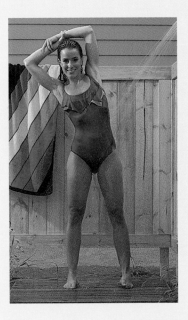

similar to that of a mechanic: "We help get the malfunctioning parts back in running order, but maintaining the machine is your responsibility."

WHY'S THIS OSTEOPATH LOOKING AT MY SPINE?

An osteopath is a trained medical doctor. Like an M.D., an osteopath can diagnose, perform surgery and prescribe medications. Unlike most M.D.'s, osteopathic physicians focus special attention on the role of the musculoskeletal system in maintaining—or disrupting—your overall health.

"Pain is a symptom of disruption. Something's wrong in your body, or you wouldn't be feeling the pain," says Dr. Hruby. "The original insult to your body may have come from an injury, accident, chronic stress, even organic disease."

Your body reacts to this insult in the same way you would: It gets uptight. "You develop secondary disorders, beginning with restricted joint movement and moving to muscle spasms. This upset in your muscular system is associated with changes in other systems throughout your body."

Your lymphatic and circulatory systems, for example, operate less efficiently around the tensed muscles. Toxic substances, including lactic acid, build up, increasing the muscles' misery. Eventually, your nervous system, noting the anarchy, signals the brain that something's rotten in the state of your muscles. The result? Your brain acknowledges the problem by having you feel pain.

"Our goal is to renormalize the muscular system," explains Dr. Hruby. "Manipulation is the key." Depending on where and how your muscles are affected, this manipulation could involve direct pressure that is similar to, though more forceful than, massage.

Supervising the patient's prescribed isometric exercises and range-of-motion stretches or actually moving the affected muscles with their hands are all part of the osteopath's arsenal.

"Through manipulation," Dr. Hruby continues, "we can restore motion within the joint and relieve the reflex muscle spasm. This allows blood and lymph to return at full force to the muscle and the joint. The circulatory and lymphatic systems are thus returned to normal functioning."

Your nervous system, recognizing the normalizing of relations, lets your brain know you no longer need to feel pain. "Our expectation is that, from this point on, the body can heal itself. When it doesn't have to deal with all of its systems being in revolt, the body can efficiently regulate itself and deal with most problems, including illness, stress or injury."

The osteopath's role is thus to relieve you of the symptom of pain, he concludes. Your job is to see to it that the pain doesn't recur. "I can help you to help your body heal itself. But from then on, you take over. You must work with your body,

Is "Rolfing" Massage Painful?

Don't avoid Rolfing just because you're afraid it's too painful. The deep muscle massage named after its inventor, the late Ida Rolf, Ph.D., isn't so bad—and it could be an answer to your agonizing chronic pain.

"I was pleasantly surprised," said a woman after her first session. "I felt some discomfort, but it never lasted more than 10 seconds. And it wasn't a sharp pain—just some twinges like bumping your funnybone."

Rolfers stroke clients' muscles with their fingers, knuckles and elbows to "loosen and lengthen" stiff muscle coverings and knead the body into perfect shape. According to Carole Lewis, Ph.D., co-director of Physical Therapy Services in Washington, D.C., the technique is similar to some of her methods and worth a try for people in chronic pain, except for the elderly, who may not respond well to the treatment. Richard Stenstavold, managing director of the Rolf Institute, says a series of 10 sessions may help others with whiplash, sciatica, scoliosis (twisted spine) or lower back trouble. So ask your doctor about Rolfing for pain relief. A list of Rolfers is available from the Rolf Institute, P.O. Box 1868, Boulder, CO 80306.

ensuring that you get adequate exercise and proper nutrition. In other words, you must become your own mechanic, working constantly to keep your body as fine-tuned as possible," says Dr. Hruby.

PHYSICAL THERAPY: PUTTING YOURSELF IN THE HANDS OF A PRO

If you need some help with this fine-tuning—if parts of you hurt and you need help in making the pain stop—consider another kind of therapist, the professional physical therapist. Physical therapists, according to Carole Lewis, Ph.D., co-director of Physical Therapy Services of Washington, D.C., are "trained health professionals who work with people's bodies to help them achieve maximum functioning. We also work with the patient to educate him about proper, health-promoting lifestyles. Effective physical therapy is a cooperative effort between patient and therapist."

If this sounds strikingly like the definition that massage therapists and osteopaths offered of their professions, it should. Again and again, these professionals sound the one all-important theme: Though they may perform the initial work of helping you heal your body, after that the control of pain is your job.

In 42 states, you need a physician's referral to be treated by a physical therapist. And in all states, your doctor (whether he's an osteopath or an M.D.) is a good place to start if you're considering physical therapy. He can tell you whether the therapy could benefit you and can also refer you to a qualified therapist.

Physical therapists, unlike osteopaths, are not physicians. They cannot diagnose the cause of your pain nor can they prescribe medications or perform surgery.

These restrictions are just fine with Steven Wolf, Ph.D. A licensed physical therapist and associate professor of rehabilitation medicine at Emory University School of Medicine, he believes that, "the best way to help people in pain is with the most conservative methods possible.

"Once you start operating on a patient to 'relieve' his pain, you significantly reduce the chance of the patient's *ever* being free of pain," he says. "And, of course, drug dependence is never a good way to deal with the problem."

MANY TREATMENTS FOR MANY PAINS

What physical therapists can do—and do well—is help relieve your pain with hands-on healing. Both massage and manipulation are in their repertoire. They also use heating pads, ice cubes, whirlpools, psychology and encouragement in their ongoing battle against pain.

"The treatment modalities that we use on any given patient depend on that person's needs," Dr. Wolf explains. "Different kinds of pain require different treatments."

Acute pain, for example, such as would accompany a sprained or torn muscle, requires quick application of cold. "You generally don't want to use heat on an acute injury, because heat draws extra blood to the area and promotes additional swelling," explains Gerald M. Aronoff, M.D., director of the Boston Pain Center at Spaulding Rehabilitation Hospital and the North Shore Pain Center at J.B. Thomas Hospital in Peabody, Massachusetts.

Cold, on the other hand, has several beneficial effects. First, it acts as a much-needed local anesthetic by numbing sensation in the area where it's applied.

It also acts as a counterirritant by loading your nervous system with too much sensory information. Your nerves can send messages to your brain, telling it, for example, that your sprained ankle hurts. But if you ice the ankle, the nerves also try to carry information saying that it is cold. With both types of impulses crowding the same path, the sensations that reach the brain are weaker. You feel less pain (see "Closing the Gate of Pain" on page 2).

Even more directly, cold relieves pain by preventing or reducing swelling. It does so by constricting the small vessels in the injured area and keeping them from bleeding. It also inhibits the body's release of hista-mines, substances that promote inflam-mation and pain.

HOME TECH

What kind of fancy technology is necessary for cold treatment? "You do need a freezer," admits Dr. Aronoff. In his practice, he freezes water in empty margarine tubs. Then he uses the tubby slabs of ice to massage the sore area.

"Ice massage involves rubbing the skin, directly, in a circular motion, with the ice. The patient's skin will first feel cold, then it will seem to burn, then ache and eventually become numb."

The whole procedure takes about 5 to 10 minutes. The pain relief lingers for anywhere from 30 minutes to 4 hours. "I have many patients who tell me that, if they massage their painful back or joints before bed, they can sleep without tran-quilizers. Many of them couldn't do that before we taught them ice mas-sage," says Dr. Aronoff.

Ice massage can be as effective in your own home as in a therapist's office, he adds. But you should always see your doctor before initiat-ing any home treatment.

In some cases, heat may be the treatment of choice, especially to help heal injuries after the acute stage is past. Whether this heat takes the form of a heating pad, a heat lamp, a dip in a warm whirlpool or a warm, wet towel wrapped around the affected limb is immaterial.

"Heat is heat," shrugs Dr. Weiner. "In any form, it's most useful two to three days after an acute injury or to combat certain kinds of chronic pain, such as arthritis."

Heat draws blood to the heated area. "One of the best things you can do for almost any injured or painful area is to give it more blood," Dr. Weiner says. The blood gives an extra boost to the body's attempts to heal itself.

"No matter how heat is applied," he adds, "an important consideration is safety: You want to heal the hurt,

not burn the patient's skin. If it hurts, stop treatment," says Dr. Weiner.

This caution is important to bear in mind, because almost all physical therapists stress that their methods can and should be adopted for home use. When people success-fully relieve their pain at home, Dr. Lewis says, "Great! Keep it up. If ice or a heating pad helps you, use it."

WORK OUT YOUR PAIN

The same do-it-yourself attitude applies in the case of therapeutic exercises. These exercises, done under a therapist's watchful eye, are another of the keystones of any physical therapy program. The first step is a realistic attitude on the part of all participants.

"We don't tell people in chronic pain that we're going to make their pain any better," emphasizes physi-cal therapist Phil Dunphy. "We give them exercises and increase their functional capacity. After a while they can do more than they could before, so to my mind they're better."

At Dunphy's Red Bank, New Jersey, rehabilitation center, the emphasis is on how well the pain patient will eventually feel, not on how poorly he may feel now. He's not treated like an invalid. He gets a towel and a locker key, just like the athletes and others who use the facility for aerobics or weight training.

"Psychologically that's impor-tant," says Dunphy. So important, in fact, that at one point he had to replace the facility's stainless steel whirlpool—and its institutional, hospital-ish feel—with a fiberglass version that looks more like a hot tub transplanted from Malibu.

The exercise programs, too, emphasize what the patients can do, often in spite of what they *think* their limitations are. "We try," he says, "to slowly get them to move the parts that hurt." After a few weeks of gentle moving, most patients—even those who feared paralysis if they exercised at all—start to feel better.

The work can be tedious and exasperating for both patient and

Phil Caruso
Edison, N.J.
Healing Method: Exercise

For someone less physically active than Phil Caruso, the car accident could've been even more tragic. And it was no picnic for him.

There he was, cruising along the New Jersey Turnpike at a steady 55 miles per hour when suddenly his hand was spraying crystals into the air from the shattered windshield and his head was reshaping the dash. His injuries, which included serious lacerations of his hand and lips, a broken collarbone and cheekbones, caved-in teeth and a dislocated jaw, only cost Phil a 4-day hospital stay. But even though the injuries healed, Phil's life was drastically changed.

Chronic pain set in: "Every day I'd wake up and there'd be a new pain. Before the accident I had been very active in all types of sports. But afterward, one day I couldn't run, the next day I couldn't play basketball. Then the pain became more specific—my lower back, my hand, my shoulder."

The lower back pain immobilized Phil. When he realized that "a different lifestyle lay ahead," he became very depressed. Then one day, he realized he had "two choices—either keep on trying or give up." Phil kept trying. His passion for sports had taught him to "go that extra yard."

But at times it seemed that no amount of determination could stop the pain that stalked him. It was while laboring—more like agonizing—through a workout in a local health club that Phil met the man who would "change my whole outlook"—Rick Misiura, a physical therapist from Raritan Valley Physical Therapy Associates, Edison, New Jersey.

In addition to other physical therapies, Rick showed Phil a series of rehabilitative

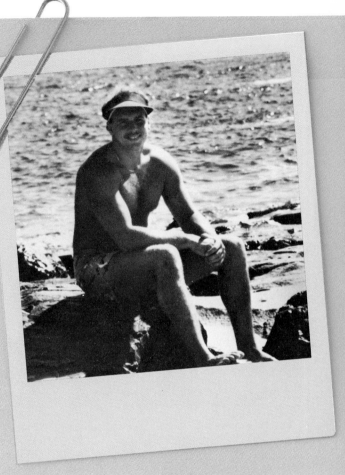

exercises that would ease the pain. "It was the exercise that helped the most," says Phil. In a few months the pain had decreased dramatically and at last Phil was more than a mere shell of his former athletic self. A year and a half after meeting Rick, he says, "I can do just about anything, though I don't like to push it yet. If I wanted to I could play a game of basketball, but I mostly swim, about 2½ miles per week, and do aerobic exercise."

Phil thinks the hour-long session of stretching and bending exercises he tries to do every day will bring him close to being 100 percent rehabilitated in another year.

He still has his bad days—usually when he skips his exercises for too long. But as with many chronic pain sufferers, Phil measures his relief relatively: "My worst days now are like my best days before I met him."

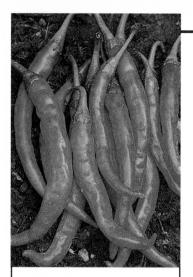

"Flame" Tames Pain

One painkiller may be found inside your favorite Mexican food. Capsaicin, the substance in chili peppers that sets your mouth on fire, takes the flame out of inflammation—in animals, at least, says Jon D. Levine, M.D., of the University of California at San Francisco.

"The principle at work is that capsaicin eventually lessens the ability of pain fibers to respond to the painful stimulus," says Dr. Levine. It's the same factor that lets people build a tolerance to fiery chili peppers. However, more research is needed before spicy food is recommended for pain relief in humans.

therapist. But it's worth it. "We're not training athletes here. We try to make people stronger and give them more ability. Exercise," Dunphy concludes, "is one of the few things they can do to really take charge of their lives."

This take-charge attitude can—and should—be translated into your at-home fitness program. Physical fitness is essential, believes Dr. Wolf. "The level of your physical fitness profoundly affects your ability to fight pain," he says.

Being in good shape means you're less likely to get in a situation in which you cause yourself pain in the first place. A well-conditioned body can better withstand the sudden, inappropriate movements that might otherwise cause sprains, strains and pains.

If you're already in pain, the fitter you are, the better you'll be able to cope, Dr. Lewis adds. "Athletes are out of the hospital after surgery more quickly than people who have 'rested up' prior to their operation," she explains. As long as you recognize your own limits, an exercise program is one of the best ways to ward off pain.

"Expect to spend at least 14 weeks getting in shape," she emphasizes. "Don't work too hard, too fast. Don't get discouraged and don't quit! Three and a half months isn't long to spend when you remember that what you're doing will change your life, for the better, forever."

Of course, see your doctor before beginning any exercise program. If, after receiving the doctor's blessing, you're still uncertain where to begin, Dr. Hruby suggests contacting the local YMCA or community health organization. They often sponsor exercise programs for cardiac patients that happen to be especially good for pain patients as well. "The groups are well supervised and structured. I highly recommend them," says Dr. Hruby.

EAT BETTER TO BEAT PAIN

To achieve maximum pain relief—and also to make your exercise easier—you need to couple your exercise

regimen with good dietary habits. Begin, if necessary, by losing weight. Being overweight can make many kinds of pain worse.

"Extra pounds put extra stress on the spine and joints," Dr. Wolf points out. "Plus, obesity demonstrates a fundamental disassociation from your body. This, of course, is unhealthy."

The problem seems to be that many people in pain have "given up" on their own bodies. "Pain patients in my practice eat an even worse diet than the average American," explains C. Norman Shealy, M.D., director of the Shealy Pain and Health Rehabilitation Institute in Springfield, Missouri. "They've already decided that health is not worthwhile or is impossible and they simply don't pay much attention to good nutriton."

This attitude is, of course, self-defeating; being healthy and being pain free are intimately related. If you need help improving your diet, contact your local hospital's physical therapy departments, which usually have resident nutritionists or dietitians who work closely with pain patients, helping them plan healthy menus and lose weight. These professionals can be an excellent resource. Hospitals often sponsor weight-loss groups or offer nutrition lectures as well.

But, you may ask, with so much else, especially pain, on my mind, why should I worry about what I eat? Because, as Harold Gelb, D.M.D., author of *Killing Pain without Prescription*, stresses, "without a balanced diet, the body can't be the self-healing, healthy system it was meant to be."

YOU AND YOUR BODY: PARTNERS IN THE FIGHT AGAINST PAIN

Remember, the point of all these therapies is to help you heal yourself. All of them aim to empower you, because "even acute pain, such as a sprained ankle, leaves you feeling vulnerable and out of control," says Dr. Weiner.

"Chronic pain," he adds, "is

Amino Acid for Pain Relief

You've seen tryptophan sitting on shelves in health food stores for years. But did you know that doctors recently started using the amino acid as a painkiller? Studies have shown that tryptophan can be remarkably useful in treating migraine, backache, neuralgia and dental pain. "It's now one of my top 10 techniques for pain relief," says C. Norman Shealy, M.D., director of the Shealy Pain and Health Rehabilitation Institute in Springfield, Missouri.

Tryptophan is a substance that turns into serotonin, a chemical messenger that sends information to nerves in the brain. Serotonin regulates sleep, increases pain tolerance and relieves depression partly by activating beta-endorphins, the brain's natural opiates. According to Dr. Shealy, 80 percent of chronic pain sufferers have lower-than-normal levels of the chemical—an imbalance that tryptophan can cure.

Turkey, peanuts, tuna, chicken, beef and dairy products all contain large amounts of tryptophan, but Dr. Shealy says adding them to your diet isn't enough. He prescribes tryptophan for his patients, starting with a megadose of 8 to 10 grams per day, then tapering down to 3 grams per day after a month. He says that eventually a daily dose of 500 milligrams keeps his patients pain free.

He also insists they take 100 milligrams of vitamin B complex while on the therapy. "Without it," Dr. Shealy warns, "tryptophan is ineffective and can make you mentally confused." (Dr. Shealy uses these substances in large, druglike doses. They're *not* for self-medication. In fact, don't take tryptophan—or any other supplement—without your doctor's approval and supervision.)

Dietary changes are also necessary to ensure tryptophan's effectiveness, says Samuel Seltzer, D.D.S., director of Temple University's Maxillofacial Pain Control Center in Philadelphia. Normal diets contain all the necessary amino acids and force tryptophan to fight for space in the bloodstream, so Dr. Seltzer prescribes a low-protein, high-carbohydrate diet that limits the other amino acids. His patients avoid red meats, cheese, eggs, butter and oils while under treatment. "If people stay on the diet and use tryptophan, the results are excellent," Dr. Seltzer says. "But if they cheat on the diet, the pain comes back."

Although tryptophan is nearly free of side effects, some users do experience mild nausea and diarrhea. People with ulcers, kidney disease or diabetes should avoid the treatment. Again, anyone interested in using tryptophan should see their doctor before taking the supplements.

worse. It disrupts your whole life. People in chronic pain typically feel there's nothing they can do to help themselves."

But, as you now know, there is. Visit one of these therapists, or follow their programs on your own (having first, of course, checked with your doctor). Most important, emphasizes Dr. Weiner, "enter into partnership with your body." Only then can you begin, at last, to take control of your pain instead of allowing it to control you.

9

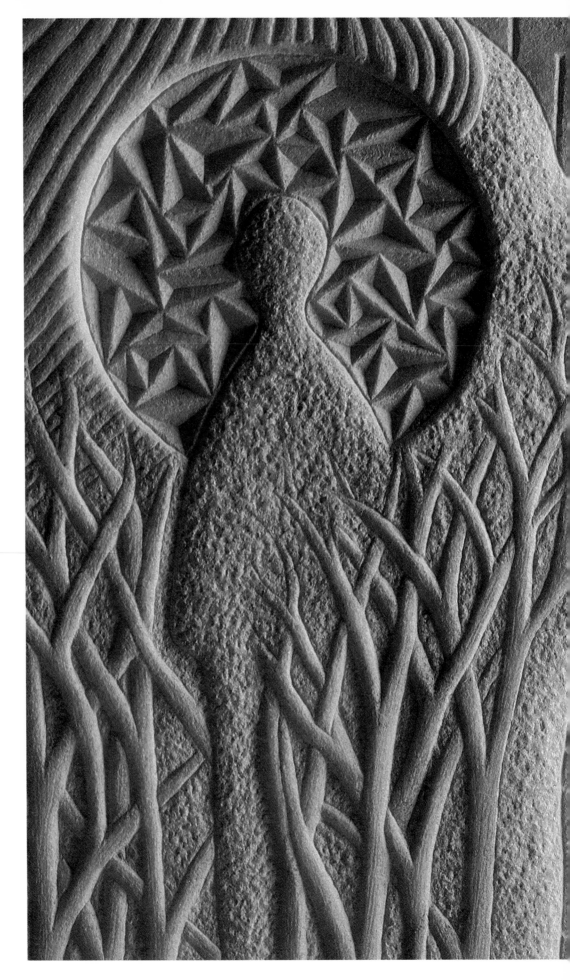

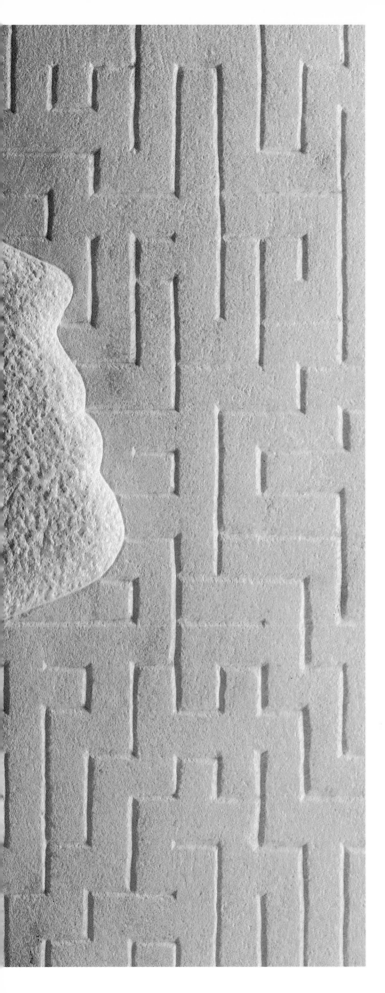

The Power of Your Mind

Biofeedback, hypnosis and visual imagery let your brain win out over pain.

W hile it's true that if a doctor says your pain is "all in your head," you ought to look for a new doctor, don't turn on your heels if someone says your pain *relief* is all in your head.

Doctors, psychologists and other experts are rediscovering what was common knowledge before scientific medicine brushed many traditional treatments aside: The *mind* can be the most powerful tool people have to fight disease—painful disease.

And advances in medicine are making fighting pain with the mind—through visual imagery, hypnosis and biofeedback—easier to do and easier to understand.

Visual imagery is a pain- and disease-fighting tool used at places such as the Simonton Cancer Institute in Pacific Palisades, California. This technique helps people visualize their body's inner workings to help them relieve pain.

Hypnosis has established itself—not as a parlor trick but as an important tool to free people from their painful chains. Many people who suffer limiting, debilitating pain find that hypnosis gives them relief when nothing else works.

Biofeedback lets people actually control their bodies' responses to painful injury and disease. With it people monitor their blood flow, heart rate, brain waves and other body functions that previously seemed beyond control. Diminished pain is the result.

There is no doubt that these medical techniques work for many people—without the side effects, astronomical cost and disruption common to many other medical treatments. And here's how they do it.

SEE THROUGH YOUR PAIN

When silver-tongued salesmen, sidewalk hustlers and fairground barkers say "what you see is what

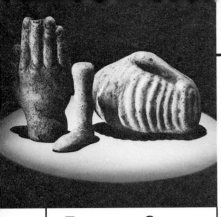

Images from the Past

Modern medicine uses high-tech tools like computers to help people ease their pain with visual imagery, but the technique is nothing new. Even the ancients used imagery: They imagined "transferring" pain and illness in diseased body parts to inanimate replicas, like the hands above. American Indians visualized their pain being sucked away by wooden pipes and used gourd rattles to "draw out" disease demons and the pain that went with them.

you get," your gut reaction is probably instant mistrust. Surprisingly, many doctors are adding a new twist to the old carney theme and using it to take the pain out of disease and injury. What your mind can see, they say, is what your body can become.

So what are highly respected doctors, and psychologists as well, doing offering this spurious-sounding sales pitch?

They're relieving pain with a technique called visual imagery. It's a new way of looking into yourself. And the end product is the relief of maladies as far-ranging as toothache, back pain and the pain of heart disease and cancer.

Just ask Margo.

By age 43 Margo had already undergone a radical mastectomy of her left breast in an attempt to stop the onslaught of potentially deadly cancer and its all-encompassing pain. Her biggest fears were realized when further tests showed the cancer had metastasized—minute cancer cells that had been missed during the initial surgery had spread throughout her system and were destroying other parts of her body. The pain was devastating and her future was bleak.

Then Margo's doctors taught her a new cancer-fighting technique: visual imagery. They told her that instead of giving in to her pain and disease she should visualize what she wanted to have happen in her body.

As she lay in her hospital bed she rolled "films" in her mind; she had private screenings of her personal war with pain and disease. She would run one movie over and over. In it the cancer cells that overran her body, causing such excruciating pain, were sickly, weakened, renegade soldiers forced in the face of a greater power to desert the battlefield that was her body. Her own white blood cells—the immune system's first line of offense and defense—were knights in shining armor on powerful white chargers, armed with lances and closing in for the kill. She visualized the chemotherapy her doctors gave her as backup foot soldiers ready to deal to the death with any straggling renegades and swiftly dispatch them from her body.

The visualization turned out to

be a personal box-office hit.

Within two months Margo was out of the hospital and her cancer was in full remission. She no longer needed to visualize a war within her body—there wasn't one.

Margo's battle against painful disease is not as unusual as it may sound.

"The imagery concept is far from new," says Dr. David Bresler, director of the Bresler Center Medical Group in Santa Monica, California. "Even in the 16th century physicians used the therapeutic effects of music to soothe people and instill mental images which could be used to treat painful ailments like arthritis."

These days an ever-growing number of doctors are recognizing that a single mental picture can be far more potent than other, more "sophisticated" treatments. They're beginning to use positive images to help their patients heal themselves, says Dr. Bresler.

"For example," he says, "a patient can be taught while sitting in a dentist's chair to stop his or her gums from bleeding by creating a vivid image of that actually happening. Several dentists have reported that when they asked their patients to *imagine* that freezing-cold ice was being applied to their bleeding gums, the patients reported that the area soon became numb. In addition, the blood vessels constricted and the bleeding stopped.

"In a similar way, the effectiveness of medications can often be enhanced through imagery. A patient taking antibiotics for a painful ear infection can be taught to imagine that the blood vessels nourishing the ear are becoming dilated. This may permit more blood—and a greater concentration of the antibiotic—to flow into the ear, hastening the healing process and ending the pain," says Dr. Bresler.

TEST YOUR IMAGERY POWER

The power of therapeutic self-imagery rests on your own ability to visualize your pain and guide it to a state of wellness.

Imagery works, says Dr. Bresler, because with it you communicate directly with your subconscious mind.

Barry Kennedy
Los Angeles, Calif.
Healing Method:
Visual Imagery

Barry Kennedy (a pseudonym) was a track star and a state championship swimmer in high school. In his teens he always had the feeling that nothing was physically above him. Just ¼ inch shy of 6 feet tall and 175 pounds of solid muscle, Barry had one of those invincible bodies that just won't quit.

Then, just before his 20th birthday, the twinges of pain started.

"It wasn't acute, stabbing pain; it was more like a dull ache—the sort of pain that you can forget about if your mind's occupied. It was a nagging pain, but I wouldn't have described it as debilitating at that point. The only real difficulty I found was bending to get in and out of an automobile," recalls Barry.

Over the next 5 years the pain spread to his chest and shoulders and into his hips and legs. Finally it began to strike unpredictably in knifelike spasms acute enough to freeze him in agonizing contortions for seconds or even minutes.

His doctor's diagnosis left him stunned. "You mean I'm going to be a cripple for the rest of my life?" asked Barry when told he had ankylosing spondylitis, which causes a gradual degeneration and fusing of the joints between the spinal vertebrae.

For the pain, he was told to take aspirin, which has both anti-inflammatory and analgesic powers. And he took additional anti-inflammatory drugs like indomethacin. The doctor's prognosis was simple: "Nothing will halt the advance of the disease, but if you keep active and mobile the chances are the spine will fuse in a near-normal position and you'll avoid the long-term crippling effects."

Then, through a medical journalist colleague, Barry was introduced to visual imagery. "Look, at this point I was at the bottom of the physical barrel, and I thought that if this had worked for cancer patients, at least I could give it a shot."

David E. Bresler, Ph.D., of the Bresler Center Medical Group in Santa Monica, encouraged Barry to draw images of his pain—his spine in an ever-tightening vise, knives and daggers that would stab violently into his back. The object of the artwork was to give both Barry and Dr. Bresler a concrete illustration of the pain problem that Barry could use to make mental visual imagery.

"I also found that concentrating on mental images of my back X rays helped me focus in on the problem. I could see the raggedy-looking joints of my spine and imagine that they were supple and smooth," Barry explains.

He was then taught an imaging technique that enabled him to "shift" the pain. "I would first concentrate on moving it from the middle of my back to my left side, and then up to my arms and down to the hand. Once I had moved it into the hand I pushed it along to my little fingertip. The little ache I now had in my fingertip was nothing. I use this method most days now, and it works," he says.

Today Barry still takes medication to control the inflammation but doesn't need any pills for pain—there's hardly any left. "If you'd asked me 6 months ago to tie a pair of shoelaces in the morning I'd have said you were crazy, but now I play racquetball every morning before work. Imagery has meant a whole new lease on life for me. It may be mind over matter, but it works." says Barry.

This "inner mind," it appears, cannot always appreciate the difference between something that actually happens in the body and something that is vividly imagined. You can prove this to yourself.

Sit in a chair, relax and create a vivid picture of the following scene in your mind.

You are climbing the outside of a skyscraper, pulling yourself up window ledge by window ledge. You reach the 90th floor and look down; the street below is filled with tiny cars and dots of people. All you hear is the constant shrill whistle of the wind that whips through your clothes. Suddenly you slip. You hang for your life by the tips of your fingers. They turn white from lack of blood. You look down and the city spins around you.

If someone were to measure your blood pressure, pulse and adrenaline while you visualize this, the levels would soar. You can feel it yourself in your body—proof that imagery is a powerful tool.

Jeanne Achterberg, Ph.D., a leading researcher and author in the imagery field, believes that exercises such as this show a definite link between imagination and the body's healing process. According to Dr. Achterberg, many medical cases support this link. Often the only explanation for people's recovery from painful terminal disease is a change in the way they see their pain.

"Something happens to cause them to begin to have a different image of themselves—not of a dying person but of a well person," she says. In her own clinical practice, Dr. Achterberg has observed people who had almost total liver failure and were as yellow as a pumpkin, yet they would be up and walking around in two weeks, while another person would have a simple diagnosis of a small breast tumor and soon be dead.

"This goes beyond physiology. You cannot die from a small breast tumor. But you can die from the working of the imagination. And from the imagination you can also gain life and health," says Dr. Achterberg.

By "seeing" yourself as healthy and pain free you can convince your mind that you are that way. In doing so, says Dr. Achterberg, you can actually beef up the immune system, stimulate painkilling endorphins and cut down on potentially deadly stress.

A NATURAL RESPONSE

Imagery can be a natural response to pain, as physicians in World War I found out. The battlefield doctors were repeatedly amazed at how badly mutilated soldiers, some whose arms or legs had been blown off, frequently lost very little blood and felt no pain. By rights, many of the injuries should have made them scream in pain, says Robert Pollack, Ph.D., of Philadelphia's Temple University, author of the *Pain Free Diet*.

Where the soldiers got these extraordinary powers was a puzzle until some doctors began to look to the mind for the answer. This was their theory: The soldiers were actually almost ecstatic to have been hit, because it meant they were still alive and wouldn't have to face the horrifying death, poison gas and carnage of the battlefield again.

Apparently they realized they were going to be all right, and therefore had a renewed will to live. They had utilized a form of imagery; they saw the future as safe and free of pain, which pulled them through.

Elmer Green, Ph.D., of the Menninger Foundation in Topeka, Kansas, tells the story of a biofeedback technician who could induce a theta (immediate presleep) brain wave state and look inside his own body with imagery techniques.

When he developed painful intestinal problems, two physicians were unable to make a diagnosis and Dr. Green suggested he try imagery and "interrogate the unconscious."

He did, and received a vivid description of his intestines, which were "thick and tough" and in them "knobby blood vessels were becoming brittle and beginning to crack."

Dr. Green confirms that he encouraged the young man to return to the doctors and tell them he had a "dream" which described his symptoms. Further tests were performed and, sure enough, the problem was diagnosed as Crohn's disease, a painful intestinal problem with

Drawing on Inner Strength

These drawings were actually made by a person suffering from chronic pain. And they weren't for an art appreciation class—they were part of medical therapy. David Bresler, Ph.D., of the Bresler Center Medical Group, in Santa Monica, California, leads his patients through "three stages of mind control analgesia" in which they draw images of their pain at its worst, when it feels the best, and how it would feel if they could control it. This gives them something concrete to work from as they use visual imagery to plot

their transformation into pain-free people. It also gives Dr. Bresler a clearer idea of the progress people make as they move from being victims of their pain to taking control of it. The technique is now widely used, says Dr. Bresler.

The drawings show one woman's perception of her pain at its worst and at its best.

some features exactly as the technician described.

MAKE IT WORK FOR YOU

Imagery is used by doctors, counselors and other therapists. But because no license is necessary to practice imagery, you want to take special care to make sure your therapist is qualified. A safe bet is to have your doctor recommend someone, or go to

a therapist who is affiliated with a multidisciplinary pain clinic (see chapter 11) or contact the American Association for the Study of Mental Imagery, c/o Jack Connella, Ph.D., 111 North Cienega Boulevard, Beverly Hills, CA 90211 for the name of a professional imagery therapist in your area.

Imagery therapy may or may not be covered by health insurance, says Dr. Bresler, depending on the qualifications of your therapist and the policies of your insurance company.

Hypnosis Cools Burns

Those victims of severe burns who are hypnotized to believe they feel cool, calm and pain free suffer less, recover faster and have less inflammation (and thus less tissue damage), reports Dabney Ewin, M.D., a surgeon and psychiatrist at Tulane University in New Orleans. Other researchers say hypnosis also reduces the need for painkillers such as Demerol. Hypnosis works best when it is induced within 2 hours of the burn.

When the therapy is done by a doctor or psychologist, an insurance company may not question your claim, especially if the imagery is listed as "psychiatric therapy" or "psychological counseling." The only way to be absolutely sure if you are covered is to check with your insurance company and your therapist.

Once you start your therapy, keep in mind that the vividness of your own imagination, together with the absolute will to see it work, is the key to success with visual imagery. "I'm not saying it is for everyone, or that anyone can do it. It takes 100 percent commitment," says Dr. Achterberg.

When your body is in pain, that commitment is worth the effort.

HYPNOSIS FOR PAIN

Hypnosis once belonged to the world of the occult. But then, so did medicine.

Today, numerous medical schools teach hypnosis, and doctors, dentists and psychologists use it to treat patients with burns, migraine headaches, cancer pain, shingles, arthritis and low back pain.

Still, many people hang on to the traditional image of what hypnosis is: The man with a goatee and a thick Austrian accent holds the chain that lets the pendulum swing in front of your eyes. The shades in the room are drawn and all that is keeping the room any brighter than a tomb is a flickering candle. The flame reflecting off the shiny pendulum soothes you into a state of servitude. "You are growing sleepy," says the hypnotist, his accent thick and hard to decipher. "Soon you will obey my every command."

This is many people's idea of hypnotism. But it is really only the myth of hypnosis. The truth is a bit more mundane.

MAY I HAVE THIS TRANCE?

Before he can treat pain, a hypnotist has to put his patient into a relaxed state. He can use a variety of induction techniques. Typically, he will speak to the patient in a gentle, rhythmic voice. He might ask the patient to close his eyes. Then he will soothe the patient into a state of complete relaxation, using his voice and suggesting visual images.

"I ask him to visualize a stairway," one hypnotist says. "I ask him to walk down the stairs with me, one step at a time, while I count from 20 to 1. With each step, I tell the patient that he is becoming more and more relaxed, and that by the time we reach the bottom of the stairs, his conscious mind will be asleep."

If all goes well (and it may not until the second or even the third session), the patient will have slipped into a hypnotic trance.

The trance is not, however, the "zombie state" that many people imagine. "People think that in a trance a person will do anything that the hypnotist wants him to do. None of that happens in real hypnosis," says Jeanine LaBaw, Psy.D., of Denver, who works with hypnosis and pain. "You totally maintain your own control. You won't do anything immoral. You won't take your clothes off and cluck like a chicken, unless you happen to like being the life of the party."

Once people enter a trance, a hypnotherapist enables them, in a sense, to imagine their pain away. By suggesting mental pictures at a time when the mind is especially receptive to them, the hypnotherapist can attach pain to an image and then move that image from one body part to another, or even push it out of the body, says Daniel Kohen, M.D., associate director of behavioral pediatrics at the Minneapolis Children's Medical Center.

Hypnosis helped one man overcome back pain, for example. "One of my patients, a 45-year-old executive named Henry, suffered from severe back pain," says Dr. Bresler. "But through symptom substitution [a mental technique for shifting pain from one place to another], he was able to move that pain from his back down to the bottoms of his feet." Eventually he was able to rid himself of his pain whenever it recurred by "walking it away." He imagined the pain leaving his body "and scattering on the ground as he walked along."

A very common technique called glove anesthesia has been used to reduce labor pains. An obstetrician might lead his patient to believe that her hand is numb by telling her under hypnosis that it's made of wood or stone or that it's a thick, woolly glove. He can then ask her, through symptom substitution, to transfer that numbness to her abdomen. After several sessions she will have learned to numb her belly simply by saying the word *belly*. She can then use this technique to limit the pain in childbirth.

THE ULTIMATE BEDSIDE MANNER

While these examples show *how* hypnosis works, they don't explain *why* it works. Assuming that there is no hocus-pocus involved, on what level of mind or body does hypnosis work?

One theory is that hypnosis, in a powerful way, distracts us from pain. "The explanation for suggested anesthesia," says Martin Orne, M.D., Ph.D., director of the unit for experimental psychiatry at the Institute of Pennsylvania Hospital, "must probably be sought in the profound effect hypnosis may exert on selective attention." In other words, we can use the hypnotic state to focus all of our attention away from the pain.

People can "choose to see or not to see" their pain better, says Dr. Orne. He also thinks that hypnosis can work by relaxing those in pain, diminishing their fear of pain.

Another theory is that during hypnosis the brain releases endorphins, the natural opiatelike painkillers. This theory is espoused by Paul Sacerdote, M.D., a New York psychiatrist and oncologist who has had great success treating cancer pain.

Others believe that hypnosis acts through emotions. Theodore X. Barber, Ph.D., a Massachusetts psychologist, thinks the success of hypnosis depends on the rapport that the doctor establishes with the person undergoing hypnosis. Hypnosis, he suggests, is the ultimate bedside manner.

The interplay between the hypnotist and the patient pushes aside the loneliness, anxiety and tension that makes pain so much worse.

At the heart of hypnosis, says

Dr. Barber, is the principle that pain fluctuates depending upon the way we perceive it. "Since the interpretation of pain sensations is such an important part of the total pain experience, hypnosuggestive procedures can play an important role in pain control," he says.

ARE YOU A GOOD CANDIDATE?

But supposing that hypnosis works, does that mean it will work for

---

Hypnosis Quiz

How good a hypnotic subject you will be varies from person to person. At least 70 percent of the population can be hypnotized, so chances are you're in that group. Here's a quick, informal test put together by psychiatrist Barbara DeBetz, M.D., to evaluate your own hypnotic susceptibility.

1. How would you characterize your tendency to trust people?
(a) above average   (b) average   (c) below average
2. In a situation where someone has to take control, do you prefer to take it or would you rather give control to someone else?
(a) I always let the other person take over   (b) It depends on the situation   (c) I always like to take control
3. Do you tend to absorb new information unquestioningly, or do you usually analyze it critically first?
(a) absorb naturally   (b) depends   (c) always critically analyze
4. Sit or lie down, close your eyes and imagine that your right hand has become very numb—so numb that you can hardly move it. How easy is this for you to do?
(a) very easy   (b) possible, but not easy
(c) impossible.
5. Do you get so absorbed in doing something that you almost forget where you are?
(a) frequently   (b) occasionally   (c) never

If you have all *(a)* answers, you are probably highly hypnotizable.

If you have mainly *(b)* answers, you are somewhat hypnotizable.

If you have mainly *(c)* answers, you are probably only slightly hypnotizable, or not at all.

everyone? The question, "Who is hypnotizable?" is much debated among researchers. The consensus is that there are a few people—known as "somnanbules" or "hypnotic virtuosos" —who can be hypnotized so deeply that they could undergo open-heart surgery without chemical anesthesia. At the other extreme, there are a few people who can't be hypnotized. Most people, however, can be hypnotized to a certain degree.

"Almost anyone can get into a trance state," says Dr. LaBaw. "If you're motivated to do it, and if you work on it, then you can do it. I have been using hypnosis in my practice for 14 years. In that time, only one or two people weren't hypnotizable."

But not all subjects are created equal. The better you are at letting your imagination run loose, it seems, the better your chances of being hypnotized. "The main thing is the imagination," says Stanford University's Ernest Hilgard, Ph.D., a pioneer in this field. "It means having the ability to believe that you are in a nice warm pool in the South Pacific instead of sitting in a dentist's chair having your teeth drilled."

Because imagination is so big a part of their lives, children have been found to be highly hypnotizable. "We know that children whose parents read them stories are likely to be good candidates for hypnosis. By age 12, some people lose a lot of their ability to be hypnotized," says Helen Crawford, Ph.D., who chairs the American Psychological Association's division of psychological hypnosis.

Dr. Barber suggests this instant "litmus test" to find out if a person is highly hypnotizable: "Ask someone to close her eyes and to imagine that she is holding a baby. Ask her to smell the baby, to feel the baby, to listen to the baby for a short while. Then tell her to open her eyes and *see* the baby. If she really sees the baby, she's a good candidate for hypnosis."

Motivation can be as important as imagination, especially for those who see hypnosis as the last resort for pain relief. The fact that they often focus all of their hope and attention on the doctor makes them more sensitive to trance induction. "Motivation is as important as hypnotic responsiveness in predicting the patient's ability to derive pain relief," says Dr. Orne.

HYPNOSIS AT HOME

And people can learn how to hypnotize themselves so that they can slip into a trance whenever pain occurs, without the presence of a hypnotherapist.

Self-hypnosis, which calls on the patient to say the words of induction to himself, is effective against pain in part because it offers empowerment, doctors say. It gives patients a tool with which they can fight their pain actively. In doing so, self-hypnosis reduces the sense of helplessness that is known to make pain seem worse than it might necessarily be. The best way to learn how to hypnotize yourself is to have your therapist teach you. According to Dr. Hilgard, "All good hypnotists teach self-hypnosis."

CONTROL YOUR BODY WITH BIOFEEDBACK

Delores Borough's migraine headaches had been ruining her weekends for three years. "They'd often come on a Saturday morning, which meant I'd either spend a day or two in bed or force myself to do things with my family even though I felt awful," the Topeka, Kansas, homemaker says. What's more, they were getting worse, and she was afraid she'd soon need stronger pain medication. But now Delores uses biofeedback to help her mind control her body—and her pain. Using techniques she first practiced on biofeedback machines, she wills her hands to warm up.

In less than a minute the temperature of her hands begins to rise—usually several degrees—and her pending headache is halted before it can ruin her weekend.

Ten or 15 years ago, such a mind-over-body feat would have been considered the realm of yogis and other mystics, possibly, but certainly not of Midwestern housewives. Today, though, biofeedback is becoming positively mainstream and is used by doctors across the country to control pain.

Biofeedback isn't as unusual as you might imagine. "Although most people are unaware of the process, learning always has been accomplished through feedback of one sort or another," says Richard Goldwasser, Ph.D., clinical director of the Stress Management and Biofeedback Clinic of Manchester, Inc., in Manchester, Connecticut.

"For example, in learning to hit a tennis ball, players get visual feedback about where the ball has landed and how far off the mark it was. They then modify their swing and footwork accordingly until the ball lands where they want it to. Without this visual feedback, learning would be difficult, if not impossible," says Dr. Goldwasser.

"Feedback comes in various forms," he continues. "For persons learning to drive a car with a manual transmission, the vibration and grinding of gears provide sensory feedback. As the vibrations and noise decrease, drivers know that they are learning to shift correctly. With practice, the skill becomes automatic and drivers no longer need to pay attention to the feedback that made the learning possible in the first place. It is now known that people are capable of controlling previously involuntary bodily functions in much the same way, although equipment initially is necessary to provide the biofeedback."

That's the big difference between everyday feedback and the pain-relief techniques used by medical professionals: Machines are brought in to help with pain relief.

These machines—electronic devices that look like stereo amplifiers—monitor your heart rate, skin temperature, brain wave activity and/or muscle tension so that you can see how your body responds to pain.

They let you monitor your response with digital readouts or audio tones that rise and fall as the measurements change. You can then learn what thought patterns will influence your body to do things like increase blood flow or relax muscles.

The machine is necessary because "most people are unable to detect, unaided, the small changes in responses that take place," says Neal E. Miller, Ph.D., director of the laboratory of physiological psychology at

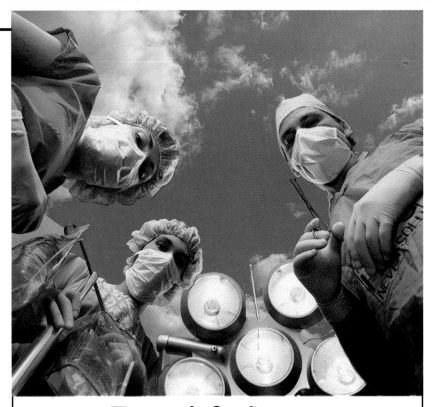

Hypnosis for Surgery

Hypnosis was the painkiller preferred by surgeons during the early 19th century, before good anesthetic drugs were developed. It baffled and mystified the doctors, but it worked.

Hypnosis is used on a smaller scale today for operations as major as open-heart surgery, as well as for more minor surgery like tooth extractions. It has even become somewhat common to see it used during childbirth. However, it is most frequently used to supplement the effects of a local anesthetic.

Rockefeller University in New York City. Dr. Miller likens trying to learn biofeedback without a machine to trying to learn the game of basketball while wearing a blindfold.

"Like the blindfolded shooter on the court, people don't get feedback and don't learn to control their responses. But modern measuring equipment can give people moment-to-moment information on many of these visceral responses and thus remove the blindfold."

The theory behind clinical biofeedback techniques says that with biofeedback you can instruct the brain to send different signals than usual to the part of the body that hurts.

If you have severe back pain

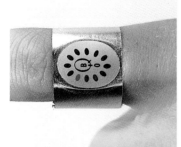

Are You Stressed?

You can use a heat-sensitive strip like the one shown above at home to give yourself a graphic idea of how to reduce your stress levels—and your pain. According to Tom Ferguson, M.D., editor of *Medical Self Care* magazine, when you attach the Velcro strip to your finger, the dots change color, one by one, around the circle. If they are brown and move in a counterclockwise direction, you are stressed. If they are blue and move clockwise, you are relaxed. To get your own home biofeedback monitor, write *Medical Self Care* Magazine, P.O. Box 1000, Point Reyes, CA 94956.

caused by muscle spasms or contractions, for instance, you would visualize the muscles relaxing. You would learn how to do this by attaching sensors from a biofeedback machine called an electromyograph (EMG) to your back muscles. The machine would give a readout of the electrical currents generated in the muscles. The therapist would explain the readout so you could see when you were relaxing the muscles.

With concentration, training and practice, you would learn how to influence these readings and to bring them as low as possible—and relieve the pain. The goal would be to become so natural at doing this that you wouldn't need the machine for feedback.

Biofeedback has been used very successfully in the control of headaches and migraines. Muscle tension pains (many of which are directly related to headache syndromes) also respond well to biofeedback therapy.

At the Menninger Foundation, Dr. Green, his wife, Alyce M. Green, a research scientist, and their clinical group have used diverse types of biofeedback training with over 1,300 patients with a variety of health problems, many of them painful. About 80 percent have succeeded in improving their condition.

The Greens believe that one of the keys to pain relief through biofeedback may be the voluntary release (as opposed to normal involuntary release) in the brain of potent endorphins.

Other research has shown that people can actually control their own brain waves with the aid of biofeedback machines. Neurobiologist and psychologist J. Peter Rosenfeld, Ph.D., and his colleagues at Northwestern University were able to train nine people to actually raise their pain thresholds by either increasing or decreasing a brain wave called an evoked potential (EP) while monitoring it on biofeedback equipment. The EP waves are usually not considered to be under conscious control or manipulation.

HOME BIOFEEDBACK

The beauty of learning biofeedback techniques is that once you learn

them, you no longer need to measure your response, because you'll become sensitive to how your body is performing. Thus, you won't need the machine.

Some sophisticated machines, especially those that read brain waves, can cost thousands of dollars—a little too much to spend for an educational tool. However, because no one needs to use the machines for long, most clinics will let you learn with their equipment. At the Menninger Clinic, for example, people are allowed to take home a portable machine for a short period until they feel they have met their goals well enough not to have to rely on it any longer.

Some people may still want to go out and buy their own inexpensive home units. Migraine sufferers might want a thermal (temperature) unit to practice regulating their blood flow, which can relax tight muscles and constricted vessels.

Dr. Goldwasser gives the following tips for purchasing home-use equipment.

- Keep in mind how long the manufacturer of the biofeedback machine has been established. Pick one that has a good track record.

- Make sure they have someone who will explain the machine and fix it if it breaks down. Find out if they will give you a "loaner" while the broken machine is being fixed.

- Does the machine have a built-in recharger? Some batteries are expensive, and have to be replaced frequently.

- Are the instruction books clear?

Simple biofeedback techniques may be learned in 6 to 8 hours of formal training. But more time may be needed, including practice at home.

Expect to pay about $50 per hour for biofeedback therapy. This will include the equipment.

If you have questions about biofeedback, contact the Biofeedback Society of America, 4301 Owens Street, Wheat Ridge, CO 80030, or the American Association of Biofeedback, 2424 Dempster Street, Des Plaines, IL 60016.

Imogene Dachenhausen
Topeka, Kans.
Healing Method:
Biofeedback

During her early years as a registered nurse, Imogene Dachenhausen would tell cancer patients who were in the last agonizing throes of the disease that they could control the pain with their minds. It worked for many—though she couldn't explain why—and later proved useful to her personally.

In the middle of a Colorado vacation, she fell. She spent a week in the hospital with a compression fracture of one of the upper vertebrae. For the next 6 months she lived in a back brace. Medications helped take the edge off the fierce pain, but she still suffered 24 hours a day.

"I was started on Percodan, and then 2 or 3 codeine preparations. Nalfon, an arthritis medication, didn't help a great deal, either. It just didn't occur to me at the time to utilize what I had been advocating in the past—the power of the mind to overcome and control pain," admits Imogene.

Severe depression set in as the months and years of agony and inactivity began to take their toll. "Life began to mean less to me. I'd come to the end of my tether," she says.

Then the former nurse was referred to Stephen Fahrion, Ph.D., an expert in the biofeedback laboratory at the Menninger Foundation near her home in Topeka, Kansas. "I didn't really have biofeedback on my mind, but at this point I was willing to try anything."

In 10 hour-long sessions at the Menninger lab, Imogene learned first how to utilize a small finger thermometer to raise the temperature at her fingertips. "Getting my temperature up showed me I could consciously direct my blood flow. At home I would spend an hour or so

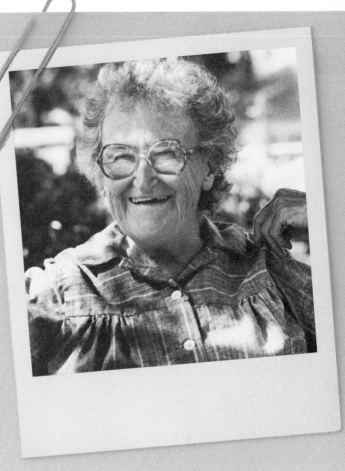

each day imagining the blood flow being directed to heal the damaged vertebra and nerves."

The next step was to familiarize Imogene with a monitoring unit that could read the tension in her back muscles. "They put electrodes on my back and I could see the increase or decrease in muscle tension on a dial. I would watch the dial move as I went into different positions, like sitting in a reclining chair or a straight-backed chair, or standing up. I was able to watch the muscles relax and I could feel the relief," she says.

Imogene almost gave up halfway through her treatment, "but something wonderful happened, and I suddenly found the pain disappearing like magic. The biofeedback worked like a charm. I sailed through the spring and summer without any pain at all. I take no medications today. There's no doubt that biofeedback has turned my life around. For the first time since the accident I am free of pain."

10

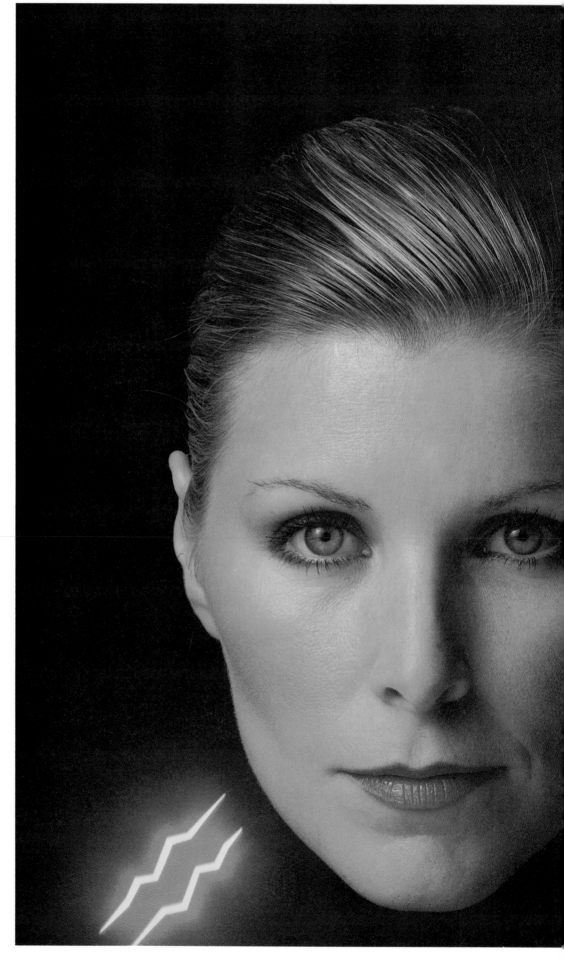

Stimulating Relief

Methods both ancient and ultra-new spark interest, controversy — and pain relief.

"If you ever want to embarrass a neurophysiologist, ask him to explain pain." That's one scientist's ironic way of pointing out that even those who've studied pain most intensively are still thrashing in the dark trying to explain it. Humankind's timeless close companion, friend and tormentor is also one of its greatest puzzles.

If how pain works is impossible to explain, how pain is relieved is just as difficult to fathom. But there have been weapons developed in the war on pain that do help control it. And in a sort of backward progression, some of these tools used to cool pain may actually lead scientists closer to an understanding of how pain functions—and ultimately to better mastery of it.

These tools seem to work in ways that are similar to pain itself. They work through stimulation— through sending or overriding messages that travel along the nerves.

These tools of stimulation have been gathered from both ends of the historical spectrum. They are our oldest and newest implements in the great battle to control pain. Among them are acupuncture, veteran of thousands of years of clinical testing, and TENS (transcutaneous electrical nerve stimulation), the little black box in the war on pain, plus a medicine chest full of modern miracles from laser light to ultrasound.

Are any of these methods for you? Can they help ease a friend's pain? What are the differences between them? And, in more detail, what are science's best explanations of how they work? Read on for a closer look at these techniques. One by one, you'll see exactly what they offer.

PINPOINT PAIN RELIEF

According to one ancient tale, acupuncture was discovered by Chinese soldiers fighting a long battle. The story says they noticed that when they received minor arrow and spear wounds, unrelated aches, colds, pains and afflictions went away.

131

Whether this story is true or not, acupuncture is unquestionably *old*. It is described in a Chinese medical text of 5,000 years ago, and stone needles believed to have been used in its practice have been found in equally ancient archaeological sites.

But time hasn't helped acupuncture gain acceptance in the West. It would be better in terms of popular acceptance if acupuncture had been discovered last year under a National Institutes of Health grant and were known as a high-tech pain reliever. Because as it is, too many people—and even physicians who should know better—see acupuncture as hocus-pocus. Witchcraft.

You can patiently explain that many doctors have found acupuncture a safe and effective pain reliever and healer. You can mention that the World Health Organization offers a long list of painful ailments from ulcers to arthritis for which it's appropriate. You can explain that it's been used and tested in a Who's Who of medical institutions that includes Stanford, UCLA and the Mayo Clinic. You can say that even an article in the conservative *Journal of the American Medical Association* has advised doctors to tell their patients that "it may well be worth a try." You can argue that the prestigious journal *New Scientist* firmly maintains it has "nothing to do with parapsychology, occult influences or 'psychic powers.'" But you'll just be tiring your vocal cords, even if you conclude with the observation that it should be obvious that a therapy that consists of sticking needles into people didn't survive for 5,000 years because it was *fun*.

ACUPUNCTURE WORKS

But acupuncture's eventual acceptance in the West as a therapy for pain and illnesses is assured, because acupuncture *works*. Doctors say that acupuncture can be effective against many kinds of headaches, many kinds of backaches, arthritis pain (particularly that of osteoarthritis), neuralgia and facial palsy. And that's only part of the list.

(We'll take a much closer look at *how* acupuncture accomplishes all these wonders as soon as we finish looking at *what* acupuncture can do.)

But it's difficult to give hard facts—statistical facts—on acupuncture.

One doctor, for instance, recalls an angry neck pain patient who left the clinic complaining loudly that the therapy hadn't helped—only to show up months later asking for treatment for tennis elbow! His neck pain, a malady he'd suffered for years, had lifted soon after he'd finished his course of acupuncture care. This kind of result doesn't lend itself to statistical analysis.

"It's not very good scientific evidence when patients tell you, 'I couldn't walk around the shopping center before, and now I can.' But it sure is convincing," says Ralph Coan,

Acupuncturists don't just poke and jab you until they find the right spots for their needles; they insert them at specific points. According to ancient Chinese theories, these points fall on lines along which your energy flows. The dots on the arm above are just a few of the hundreds of points in the body. To find them, the acupuncturist follows charts, looks for signs in the texture of the skin or uses sophisticated electrical equipment.

M.D., past president of the American Association for Acupuncture and Oriental Medicine.

Dr. Coan estimates that between 50 and 70 percent of his patients at the Acupuncture Center of Washington in Bethesda, Maryland, experience relief from many painful conditions such as osteoarthritis and back pain. Other frequently heard estimates of the percentage of people acupuncture helps range from 30 to 85 percent, depending on the condition being treated. And most of these people had exhausted all Western remedies first!

A STAINLESS STEEL PLACEBO?

Acupuncture sometimes relieves pain for years after therapy stops. In fact, sometimes it seems that acupuncture works too well and does too much. How can the insertion of simple stainless steel needles into the body possibly relieve the pain of headaches, backaches, arthritis and neuralgia, reduce swelling and inflammation, lower blood pressure, lift depression, raise the white blood cell count and improve immunity, help digestive problems, and even affect the level of fats in the blood—not to mention fight the common cold? Acupuncture's very versatility makes people suspicious and starts them thinking in terms of placebos, hypnosis, the power of suggestion.

"It's *not* one of those things that only work if you believe in them," insists Jennifer Katze, M.D., a psychiatrist who says she was skeptical and disbelieving until acupuncture eliminated the four or five debilitating colds she suffered each winter.

"Thirty percent is a standard pain relief rate for placebos," says George Ulett, M.D., Ph.D., author of *Physiological Acupuncture.* "Acupuncture often gets a 70 percent effectiveness rate. That's a pretty good placebo."

If it's not just the power of suggestion, how does acupuncture work?

The Chinese have traditionally explained it in terms of energy flow—that the needles stimulate energy where it's needed, which leads to healing.

That energy may be bioelectricity, Western doctors now say, a very real phenomenon that's measured when an EEG or brain scan is taken. Scientists confirm, too, that acupuncture points (see the illustration on page 132) can be precisely located on the skin with modern electrical equipment. But researchers have dug beyond the still-theoretical energy explanation to tell us more fully how this marvel functions.

HEALING WITH STRESS

Call acupuncture stress therapy. This phrase may best help us understand how it works. More effectively than any other method, acupuncture needles—without causing any actual harm and usually with almost no pain—convince your body that it is under attack.

As a result, endorphin levels jump. Famous as the body's own painkillers and familiar to many as the source of the "runner's high," these substances block chemical pain receptor sites in the brain.

This production of painkilling chemicals has been confirmed by studies that show that hormone-rich spinal fluid from an animal given acupuncture can raise the pain threshold when injected into an animal that hasn't had acupuncture. Both human and animal research has also shown that naloxone, a substance that blocks the effects of the endorphins, can stop acupuncture's pain relief.

These explanations easily cover acupuncture's power to limit and lift immediate acute pain. But what about the treatment's long-term pain-relieving properties? Many people get not just temporary relief, but relief that lasts for years after they stop treatment.

Scientists believe that this result is accomplished by an actual change in the nervous system. Chronic pain—pain that is unremitting by its very nature—sets up what doctors call reverberating circuits or resonating loops between the spinal cord and the brain. It's a kind of pain memory with a mechanism, says Dr. Ulett.

Acupuncture bombards those pain pathways with a different message, he says. It's sort of a super-efficient way of accomplishing the same thing you unconsciously do when you clench your jaw or fist in response to pain. It sends a different message across the circuit, which blocks the aching message.

Pain from a phantom limb is another good example of a reverberating circuit (see "Pain from Nowhere" on page 7). One woman suffered the agony of feeling her missing arm being constantly twisted and crushed behind her as her fingernails dug deeply into her palm—just as in the accident that cost her the limb, Dr. Ulett recalls. As she received acupuncture, she began to "feel" her arm resuming a normal position and her nails withdrawing from her flesh. Because of its ability to break the circuitry, acupuncture is often used successfully to treat phantom limb pain.

IS ACUPUNCTURE IN THE PHONE BOOK?

If you've decided acupuncture may be able to help you, one good way of finding a reliable acupuncturist is simply to call the American Association for Acupuncture and Oriental Medicine at (516) 627-0309. Because licensing requirements differ from state to state, this association is the surest way to check someone's credentials. Otherwise, word-of-mouth—the same method you might use to get information about doctors—may help. If you haven't been diagnosed by an M.D., be sure you are before proceeding.

A VISIT TO AN ACUPUNCTURIST

Once you've chosen your acupuncturist, you may be a little disappointed to find his or her office much like any doctor's space, with no brass gongs, smoking incense or paunchy brass Buddhas on the shelves. The acupuncturist may read your Chinese "pulses" at several places on your wrist. And you may be asked questions—how you've been eating and sleeping or if anything has been upsetting you.

Your tongue and the texture of your skin may then be inspected.

Next you'll be given a hospital robe or half sheet and asked to go into a dressing room or behind a screen to disrobe for treatment.

You're bound to be a little tense as you prepare to undergo a new procedure, but you may find your nervousness balanced by your hope that acupuncture may relieve your pain. And you will probably be reassured by the relaxed, caring and competent manner that's a sign of a good acupuncturist. Don't hesitate to ask questions.

If your condition permits, you'll probably next be asked to lie on a cushioned table. You'll be told when and where the needles are to be applied. This is where most people begin to reassess the wisdom of visiting an acupuncturist. Not many people like to be poked with needles. But you'll probably be pleasantly surprised at the lack of pain. The sterilized stainless steel needles are so thin—in some cases, only one-tenth the size of an ordinary hypodermic needle—that the sensation of being pricked is often totally absent.

What's more, it's likely that because of the endorphins and other stimulation, you'll immediately begin to feel tranquil and relaxed. Leona Yeh, Ph.D., a certified acupuncturist from Los Angeles, says that 85 percent of her patients feel calm almost immediately. Thirty percent of them even go to sleep!

"Some of our patients come in here afraid they'll end up strung out like a pincushion," Dr. Coan says. But actually, he says, it's rare for many needles to be used.

While the needles are in, the therapist may gently twirl them or even stimulate them with a very mild electrical current. You may feel a sensation of heaviness or a slight tingling. The Chinese call this feeling *te chi*, and say it's a sign that energization is taking place.

One sign of acupuncture's acceptance is that many insurance companies now cover the cost of acupuncture, which is frequently given in a series of ten or so sessions at about $35 for each session. The IRS may let you deduct acupuncture as a medical expense, so check with your accountant or local IRS office. Another stimulating therapy you may also be

Ralph Lester
Lorton, Va.
Healing Method:
Acupuncture

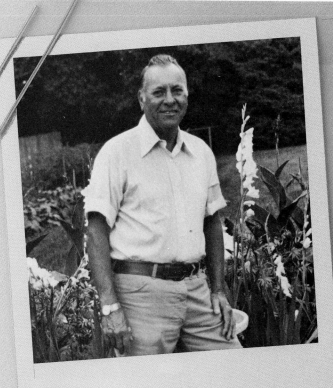

When Ralph Lester retired after more than 30 years as an offset pressman, he had something more than a gold watch and a pension. He had a bad back.

Recalling the history of the injury, he thinks he might have first hurt himself loading the huge rolls of paper into his press. Or maybe it happened while he was climbing on his machine to fix it. He never knew exactly when or how he'd done it. All he knew was, his back hurt.

After an unsuccessful course of serious pain medications and heat treatments, physical therapy at an orthopedic hospital finally brought him relief.

But then the ice storm came, his wife, Madeleine, recalls. Ralph went to work early to clear the walk so the women employees could get to their jobs safely, Madeleine says. When he fell, he cracked three ribs and reinjured his back. Unaware of the seriousness of his injury, he finished out the day at work. But by the time he got home, the pain was telling him to see a doctor.

Again, he was put on Percodan, Darvon and Tylenol with Codeine. The ribs mended, but the back pain didn't leave. He couldn't drive his car. And he had to sleep in a reclining chair. If he lay down in bed, he couldn't get up. His doctor began talking about an operation.

"I didn't think much of that," remembers Ralph. So when a news program on TV featured a segment on acupuncture and he heard an M.D. advising anyone considering a back operation to try acupuncture first, he was ready to listen. He asked his wife to find him an acupuncturist.

Ralph hurt so badly that he had to be helped to the car for the 40-mile trip from his home to the Acupuncture Center of Washington in Bethesda, Maryland.

At the center, he was examined by a doctor who looked at his X rays before offering acupuncture.

"They told me they thought they could help me, but they couldn't guarantee it," Ralph recalls. But after just 3 treatments, which he found virtually painless, he was able to resume driving. After 10 treatments, the pain in his back was gone.

The entire course of treatment cost about $350 and relieved another problem besides. The arthritis in his hands, which had become so bad he sometimes couldn't close his fingers, was so much better after the acupuncture that he began doing free-lance carpentry.

Three years after treatment, Ralph Lester is still free of pain. He recently poured the concrete foundation for an addition that he's building.

able to deduct is transcutaneous electrical nerve stimulation (TENS). While it is a modern therapy, TENS—like acupuncture—is rooted in the past.

TIME TRAVEL AND ELECTRIC PAIN RELIEF

The year is A.D. 47, and your doctor is writing a prescription. You are to stand in shallow sea water on a live black electric torpedo fish until your legs are numb to the hip. This is a sure cure, your physician, Dr. Scribonius, tells you, for the excruciating pain of your gout.

"They were essentially doing TENS there," affirms Albert Kuhfeld,

Ph.D., curator of Minneapolis's Bakken Library, which is home to a collection of electromedical devices and literature spanning two millennia.

So TENS, an increasingly popular electrical treatment that can stop pain by passing mild currents across the skin, wasn't borrowed from the future or from science fiction, after all—though it looks as though it might have been.

Today's TENS is usually given by means of a battery-operated, portable device about the size of a deck of cards. Wires connect the case to dial-regulated electrode patches taped to your skin, usually near the pain site.

And though at first its patches, wires and knobs may make you remember Frankenstein's monster being jolted to life by a current of electricity, TENS is more likely to leave you thinking of gratitude if you are a pain sufferer.

TENS units are relieving the aches and agonies of everything from childbirth to terminal cancer. Safe, practical and nonaddictive, TENS' popularity is growing rapidly. (The only people who should be wary of TENS are pregnant women, people with pacemakers, and people who are allergic to the adhesive that attaches the TENS patches to the skin.)

In a typical year, approximately 130,000 people turned TENS on to their pain. The largest number of users were chronic back pain sufferers, and many found that turning on TENS turned pain off, or at least turned it down.

TENS has become especially popular with athletes, who are often injured in the line of duty. Golfers Lee Trevino and Fuzzy Zoeller have felt the relief of TENS. Thanks to their treatments, they've been able to perform at times when they might otherwise have been sidelined.

CURRENT PAIN RELIEF FROM THE PAST

Today's TENS delivers a sophisticated and carefully modulated form of electrical therapy. But its high-tech accuracy stands at the end of a long line of hit-or-miss electrical devices,

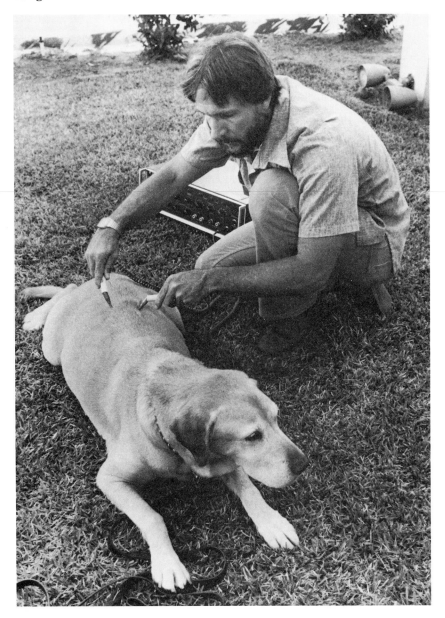

No, this man isn't trying to jump-start a dog, He's giving it a form of electric acupuncture to relieve the pain of arthritis. San Diego veterinarian Bruce Cauble, D.V.M., uses this therapy to try to control the pain and therefore reduce the amount of corticosteroids (anti-inflammatory drugs) being used.

many of which are on exhibit at Dr. Kuhfeld's Bakken Library.

Even an old-time carnival device that tested how much of a jolt fairgoers could stand provides pain relief, Dr. Kuhfeld says. After demonstrating the contraption—which for a coin allows the user to turn a dial controlling the current to a hand-clasp—Dr. Kuhfeld says he notices that his own middle-age aches and pains vanish for a few hours. He says you could even build a self-generating TENS unit from old pie plates and other household items. But to carry it with you, you'd need a large purse. You'd also need "a loyal and sturdy companion to turn the crank," he says.

Crank is the word for it. Throughout history, electricity has had periods of being fashionable, Dr. Kuhfeld says. Around the turn of the century, the mail-order giants Montgomery Ward and Sears, Roebuck sold many small, battery-operated devices for home medical treatment.

But electricity became too popular for its own good. Outlandish claims were made for its healing properties. Charlatans and quacks added electrical contraptions to their line of snake oil nostrums and promoted them as cure-alls. Sold under names such as the "Pulvermacher Electric Belt" (which had to be soaked in vinegar before use) and the "Electropoise," the gizmos falsely claimed to cure everything from athlete's foot to dandruff. As a result, electrical devices fell into disrepute with serious medical workers. The one thing they may have done well—relieve pain—was dismissed along with the bizarre boasts.

HOW ELECTRICITY TURNS OFF PAIN

Fortunately, we now know that electricity can kill pain. But whether from fish, eel, pie plate, carnival contraption or TENS, exactly how does electricity throw the switch on pain?

At least two mechanisms appear to be involved, say doctors. First, TENS can stimulate the neural system the same way acupuncture does, making the body produce its own natural painkillers. In fact, TENS electrodes are often placed over acupuncture points and one form of TENS is known as "acupuncturelike." And, like acupuncture, TENS may provide relief for some time after it has been given.

TENS may also provide relief in the same way "acoustical perfume" does, suggests Dr. Kuhfeld. An example of acoustical perfume is turning on your fan to mask the noise of your neighbors' patio party. Though the party noise is still there, all you hear is the gentle whirring of the fan. After a while, you can't even consciously hear the fan.

That's really just another way of visualizing the classic, 30-year-old gate control theory of pain, which suggests that both pain and touch impulses feed into the same neural highway. If this highway gets bumper-to-bumper with touch and pressure sensations, pain impulses can't crowd in to get to the brain.

WHY RELIEF MAY BE SPELLED T-E-N-S

Ronald Dougherty, M.D., loves TENS. It's not just that as director of the Pelion Pain Clinic and medical director of the Chemical Abuse Recovery Service at the Benjamin Rush Hospital in Syracuse, New York, he sees TENS relieve pain every day. It's not even the studies he's run on hundreds of patients to prove TENS' effectiveness to himself.

Dr. Dougherty loves TENS because he used to treat drug addicts, helping them detoxify. He soon learned that as many as 30 percent of addicts were hooked on drugs given to them by their physicians. Prescription drugs were actually causing more of the overdoses and accidental deaths seen in emergency rooms than street drugs, he learned.

But the worst came after Dr. Dougherty had helped the doctor-created addicts get free of their Dilaudid, Percodan, Demerol or Darvon habits. Then they'd turn to him and say, "Thanks for getting me off drugs. Now what are you going to do about my pain?" he recalls grimly. Now he can respond, "I've got something for you—TENS."

TENS causes no grogginess, no clouded judgment, no addiction. The worst hazard of TENS use is skin irritation at the site of the electrode pads. (One user reports, however, that the fresh juice of the aloe vera plant cleared up a rash within days.)

Another user experiences another minor problem. "Sometimes I get hung up with the wires on doorknobs or car door handles," she says.

But a more serious problem can develop if TENS is not used correctly, Dr. Dougherty warns. And that is simply that the treatment may lose effectiveness. When patients turn their units higher and higher in an effort to get more and more relief, they may defeat themselves. Tolerance to TENS can develop.

But tolerance need not happen, Dr. Dougherty maintains. One of his patients has been getting good pain relief from TENS for a decade, he says.

Using TENS at a high setting may also cause muscle contractions. (This is how commercial promoters of "passive exercise"—a system pushed as an easy alternative to a strenuous workout—perform their doubtful wonders. It is also a means used to stimulate the muscles of stroke victims and other patients, with healing results.) When jolts are this strong, a patient may wear out TENS' usefulness quickly, doctors warn.

SHOCKINGLY PLEASANT

What the usual dose of TENS feels like is a mild tingling. A higher setting may cause a pulsing feeling. Most people find neither of these sensations unpleasant.

"We've been trained to fear electricity," Dr. Kuhfeld says. "And that's right because there are some pretty powerful currents flowing behind those cords, sockets and plugs.

"But, as with the carnival device, if you can bring yourself to hold on, you discover that it doesn't hurt. You say, 'Oh, that's what electricity feels like,'" he says.

Physical therapist Julie DeVahl, an employee of the Medtronic Company, a maker of TENS machines, has another approach to patients' fears. "I don't mention electricity,"

she says. "I tell a patient, 'I'm going to put some patches on your skin that will send a signal to your nerves that will tell them to ignore the pain.'" This works, she claims, though it sometimes gets a little sticky when she has to explain how to change the batteries.

CAN YOU COUNT ON TENS?

If a physician or physical therapist prescribes TENS for pain that's been troubling you for a long time, you'll probably be given a rental unit for about a month. This will ensure that the relief that you felt in a medical setting was not just a placebo effect and that you *are* one of the estimated 70 percent of people who can be helped by electrical stimulation. (For reasons doctors don't really understand, 30 percent of people don't respond to electrical stimulation as a pain reliever.) In fact, today's everyday TENS was actually developed as a testing device to make sure patients could be helped by surgically implanted electrodes. Doctors quickly figured out, however, that TENS itself was often the best alternative for pain relief. However, for some types of chronic, unremitting pain, surgeons still choose to implant permanent electrodes in the brain or, more commonly, along the spinal column.

If you're being treated for acute pain—pain that's not expected to last—such as postoperative pain or the pain of a pulled muscle, you will also probably use a rented machine. But if your pain is chronic, and you find that the rented machine gives you relief, your medical insurance may reimburse you for the $500 or $600 cost of purchasing a unit. Check with your insurance carrier.

Dr. Dougherty would like to see TENS prescribed far more often than it is. He believes too many physicians choose to write a quick prescription rather than taking the time necessary to train patients in TENS use.

But as word spreads that TENS is safe and effective and allows you a measure of control over your own pain, more and more patients may start asking their doctors for it. You shouldn't hesitate to join them.

Barbara Kull
Minneapolis, Minn.
Healing Method: TENS

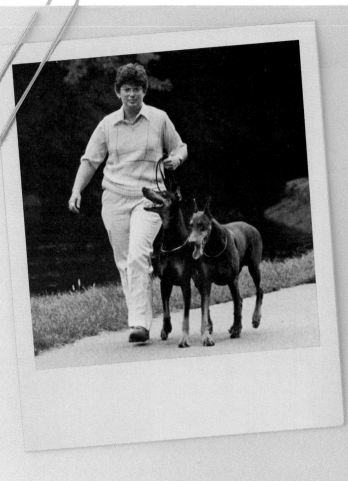

Barbara Kull used to be proud that she was a professional carpenter and floorlayer. And she was proud that she worked for the all-woman Calamity J. Construction Company in Minneapolis. She was proud, too, of an active sports-oriented lifestyle that featured horseback and motorcycle riding.

Then, in January of 1984, the speeding toboggan on which she was straddling the end seat—the spot most vulnerable to whiplash—went soaring over a 2-foot bump.

The accident fractured Barbara's 12th thoracic vertebra, pushed a bone chip against her spinal cord and left her in nearly constant, agonizing pain, pain that worsens whenever she moves. Sometimes the pain seems to fill her entire midsection. Usually it rakes across a section of her ribs and stabs behind her shoulder blade.

This is not a story about a near-miraculous recovery. Unfortunately, most chronic pain stories don't end that way. But it is a story of courage and of learning to live with pain that has radically changed her life—pain that has retreated but refuses to yield the field.

In the year after the accident, Barbara desperately went from healer to healer—3 general practitioners, 2 physical therapists, a chiropractor, an osteopath, 2 orthopedic surgeons. She hung by her feet for antigravity traction and she had normal traction. She did neck exercises and rode an exercise bike. She had cortisone injections in her joints and in her muscle trigger points.

For a too-brief, 2-week period, it seemed that the trigger-point injections given by one of the physicians were helping. They didn't. Her hopes of returning to the active lifestyle she had led as a construction worker and, before that, as a physical education teacher, were once again crushed. Even to hope for the self-sufficiency of getting herself up, dressing herself and earning a living seemed out of reach.

But then Barbara got lucky. One of the surgeons suggested TENS, and a friend gave her a unit left by a deceased relative. Barbara's insurance wouldn't have covered the $600 machine. A physical therapist taught her to use it. The first time she tried it, she was rewarded with 8 pain-free hours for the first time since the accident. Again, her hopes soared.

But Barbara's pain was not to be so easily conquered. Using TENS every day dims the pain enough for her to work as Calamity J.'s assistant general manager and be self-sufficient. But she still chafes under the sentence to a sedentary life that her pain imposes on her.

Ultrasound Finds Stress Fractures

Pain has its good points—at least according to British researchers who've discovered a simple way to help diagnose stress fractures. These tiny cracks in the bones of the lower legs and feet often plague joggers and aerobic dancers. Proper treatment depends on early diagnosis, but the fractures are notoriously hard to detect. They may not show up on ordinary X rays, but bone scans, which do reveal the cracks, are costly and bothersome. A promising alternative, however, was reported in the *British Medical Journal*. Ultrasound waves applied to the legs often pinpoint the condition. Healthy people find the ultrasound painless—only those with stress fractures feel pain.

GETTING THE RED IN

Nor should you hesitate to ask your doctor about infrared therapy. Infrared rays can penetrate clothes, hair, even a sheepdog's fur, to put healing light right where it hurts: roughly ⅓ inch beneath the skin.

"Infrared will give relief for 15 to 30 minutes for certain kinds of pain," says James Griffin, Ph.D., a physiotherapist at Ball State University in Indiana and coauthor of *Physical Agents for Physical Therapists*. It can help ease the pain of rheumatoid arthritis, torn muscles, bursitis, tendinitis and osteoarthritis.

"I'll use infrared, initially, the way a doctor uses aspirin before narcotics," Dr. Griffin says. But if the infrared doesn't relieve pain after two or three treatments, ultrasound—high-frequency sound waves—is the next step. Ultrasound is more effective than infrared at relieving pain, says Dr. Griffin, although no one is really sure how it works.

Robert Bengston, director of physical therapy at Beth Israel Hospital in Boston, suggests that in the process of heating muscles and increasing blood flow—both of which aid healing—ultrasound also stimulates nerve fibers. The fibers may then short-circuit and shut down, cutting off pain messages to the brain.

But pain relief is really only one aspect of ultrasound, says Bengston. Its primary function is to "preheat" body tissue, to loosen pain-stiffened joints and muscles so that the physical therapist can get in there and go to work. And although ultrasound may relieve pain on its own, it is more effective when combined with other therapies.

For example, Bengston worked with a patient, a 38-year-old nurse who was referred to Beth Israel for low back pain of three years' duration. She was helped by a combination of ice, ultrasound, physical therapy, TENS and exercise.

The problem, reports Bengston, was a strained muscle and a slight shift in her spinal column. He suggested she put ice on the muscle for 20 minutes twice a day for three days, then receive a week of daily ultrasound sessions followed by ultra-sound three times a week. He also recommended that she do back-flexibility exercises and use a TENS unit at home. Two weeks later, when the worst of the woman's pain had subsided, Bengston added more demanding back exercise and an overall regimen of exercises designed to help her to do everyday tasks without pain.

One week later the nurse was free of pain.

Of course, the nurse might have been pain free a lot sooner if she'd gone to Bengston immediately after her injury. Generally, Bengston reports, the most effective way to use ultrasound is to see a physical therapist as soon as possible after a painful injury or condition has developed.

For pain from newly developed problems, he suggests ultrasound treatment twice a day for two days, then once a day until the pain lets up. Less painful conditions may respond to treatments once a day for seven days, then every other day until the pain lessens. Chronic pain, he suggests, should be treated with ultrasound every other day for a period of two weeks. At the same time, the person should start a program of regular exercise.

And ultrasound can enhance the pain-relief properties of drugs such as aspirin and hydrocortisone. An ointment containing one or the other drug can be spread over painful joints or muscles, explains Dr. Griffin, and the area bombarded with ultrasound. The sound waves will drive the medication through the skin into the painful area. Then, instead of circulating through the body, says Dr. Griffin, the medication stays where it's needed—right at the center of your pain.

Luckily, ultrasound does not hurt —most people feel a slight warmth— and is covered by insurance.

But ultrasound isn't a miracle cure for a pain. Although people report pain relief, researchers are still looking for a convincing explanation. And administrators at the federal Center for Devices and Radiologic Health (CDRH) in Rockville, Maryland, express reservations about the therapy, particularly when done with units sold for home use. The units, frequently hand-held devices that emit 600,000 oscillations per second, are advertised as a treatment for bruises, sprains, strains, arthritis pain, swelling, poor circulation and even congested sinuses.

They may or may not work. But the CDRH cautions that they could be potentially dangerous if used with excessively high power by unqualified people. "If the power is high enough, you could get burned," says Bengston.

LET THE BUYER BEWARE

How can you protect yourself when dealing with technologies such as infrared, ultrasound and TENS? How can you keep from getting shafted, ripped-off, even injured?

One way, advises Deborah Downing, a registered physical therapist who has studied ultrasound devices at the University of Connecticut Health Center in Farmington, is to make certain that qualified personnel are handling the equipment. Ultrasound, for example, should be administered only by a trained physical therapist or physical therapy assistant. When you call a hospital's physical therapy department for an appointment, ask for a registered therapist who has taken any special courses related to your problem, Ms. Downing advises. If no one has, try another hospital or rehabilitation center. And keep trying until you find someone who knows what they're doing.

Another way you can protect yourself, say administrators at the federal Office of Science and Technology, is to ask the doctor, therapist or researcher for a copy of their authorization to conduct clinical investigation on the device in question. If your specialist claims it has already been approved for use by the U.S. Food and Drug Administration (FDA), ask to see the letter of approval.

When shopping for home-use devices, federal sources suggest you check the device for a certification label, which indicates that the unit meets health and safety standards established by the federal government. But even then, warns one expert, be cautious. Check the device with a qualified therapist or doctor to make certain there are no dangers.

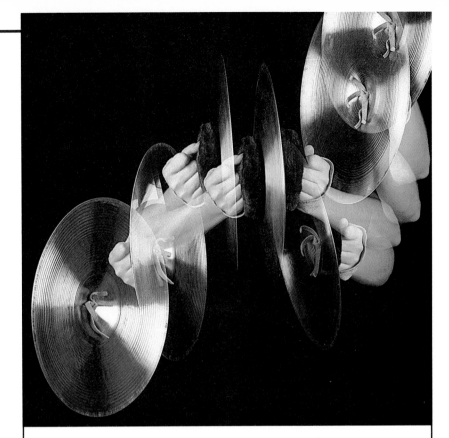

Turn Down Your Pain

If you think of pain as a sound, then chronic pain makes an awful racket. Laurence Ince, Ph.D., of the psychology service in the department of rehabilitation medicine at New York University Medical Center, asks his patients to equate their pain with sound and then turn it down.

Dr. Ince first asks patients to match their pain with the intensity of a pure tone, like those used in hearing tests. "Think about where your pain is right now," he suggests to them, "and tell me when the tone is as loud as your pain." Then he lowers the volume in 5-decibel (dB) increments. With each drop, patients are told to concentrate on decreasing their pain to match the softer tone.

At first, people often equate an 80- or 90-dB tone with their pain. "That's akin to standing on a New York City subway platform as a train roars by," says Dr. Ince. After as few as 12 sessions, however, patients usually decrease their pain significantly—often to a whisper-soft 10-dB level—or even eliminate it. And these results are long lasting. Those who do have occasional recurrences find they can sit back on their own and quickly turn down their pain as they did in the hospital.

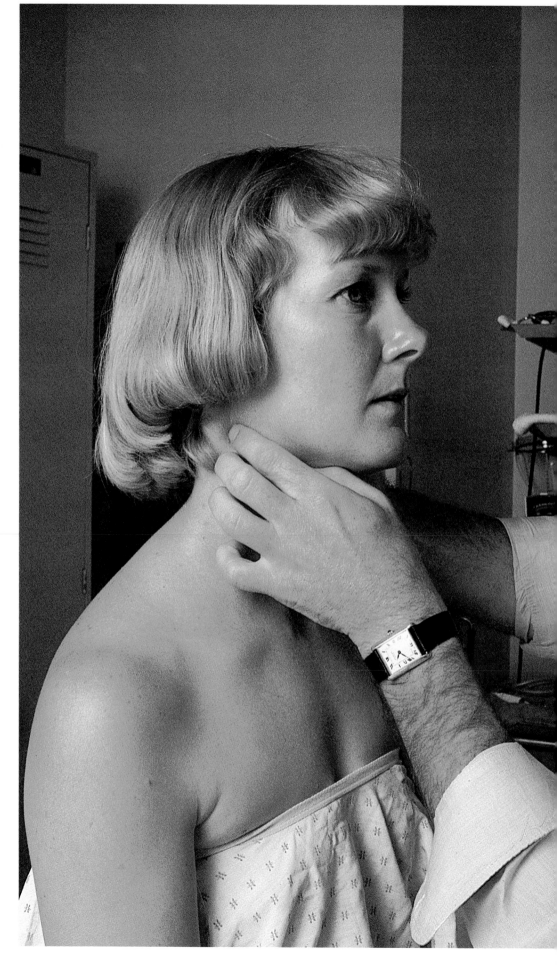

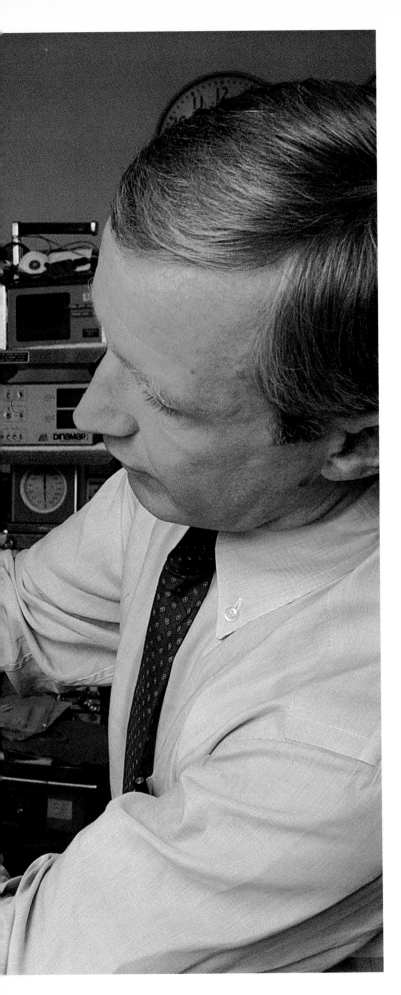

11

Visiting a Pain Clinic

This clinic—typical of dozens across the country—uses all the relief methods to help people live pain free.

Where can you turn when the pain is too much to bear and after each visit to the doctor you're left with two burning questions: "What's wrong?" and "When is it going to end?"

There's a good chance answers to both questions will be found during a visit to a pain clinic—a good pain clinic like the one at the University of Washington in Seattle, pictured in this chapter. These clinics, found in cities and towns across the country, specialize in treating people who've tried almost everything in their quest for pain relief, without success.

The University of Washington clinic was the first in the country, and it has set a standard for the others ever since. But wherever you live, there is probably a good clinic within a reasonable distance. Since many require a doctor's referral, your physician is the best source of information about quality pain clinics. The most important considerations are that the clinic be multidisciplinary, meaning it uses more than one type of treatment, and be staffed by more than one type of health professional.

Not all clinics require you to stay there. In fact, people often can be successfully treated at outpatient facilities and pain treatment centers. And don't be surprised if your doctor refers you to an anesthesiologist. According to Carol Warfield, M.D., most pain clinics in this country are run by anesthesiologists, often working with neurologists, psychologists, surgeons, physical therapists and other experts in pain relief.

At the Seattle clinic a team of doctors, psychologists, nurses and other therapists use every technique at their disposal to relieve your pain. During a typical three-week inpatient stay, you will undergo physical therapy, vocational and psychological counseling and group sessions of training in skills to manage pain and life problems caused by pain. The emphasis of these therapies is to teach people the skills they need to

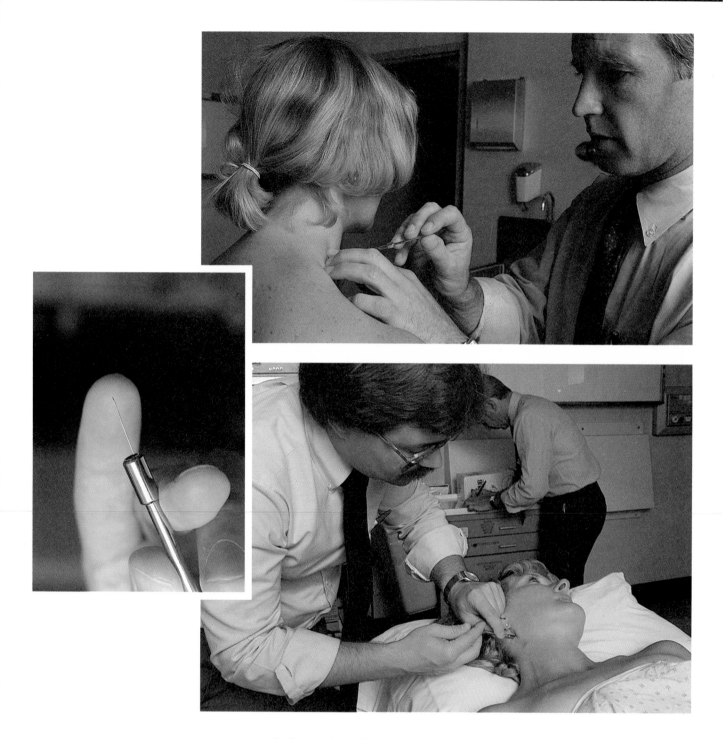

cope with their pain without using drugs. Family members and friends also are asked to visit the clinic, because they play a crucial role in how well the patient does after treatment.

The clinic sums up its aims like this: "You have a pain problem that has lasted a long time and that is interfering with your life. We are here to help you to do something about that."

In the photo on the preceding page, F. Peter Buckley, M.D., searches Sheila Bell's neck for a muscle that spasms uncontrollably, causing her great pain. On this page, left, is the Japanese needle that doctors insert into trigger points in the muscle to calm it and ease the pain, as shown in the photos above.

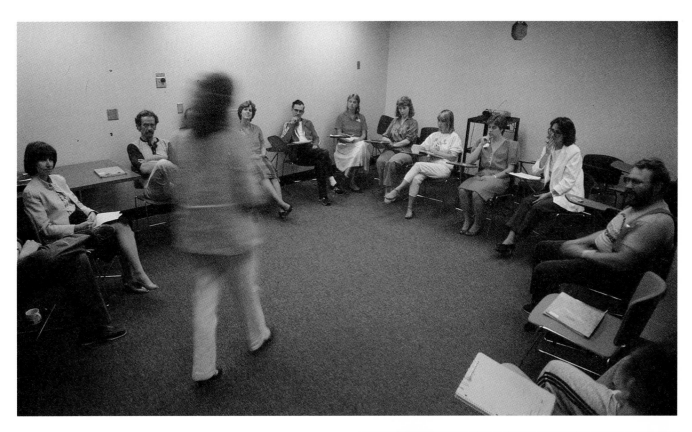

Group sessions like the one shown above are an important part of treatment at the pain clinic. Every weekday at 8:00 A.M., a group meets to learn about the many aspects of chronic pain. They learn about how the brain works to control pain, the effects of inactivity on muscles and pain, drugs taken for pain and the purpose of exercise. In the afternoon a group meets with a clinical psychologist to learn skills to deal with problems caused by pain. These may include stress management, assertion, sleep management and communication skills. Finally, in the evenings nurses conduct groups to teach relaxation techniques, help patients practice what has been learned during the day and discuss the patients' questions about their treatment.

At right, a man adjusts the level of electricity being delivered to his body from his TENS unit (see chapter 10). The gentle current offers strong pain relief.

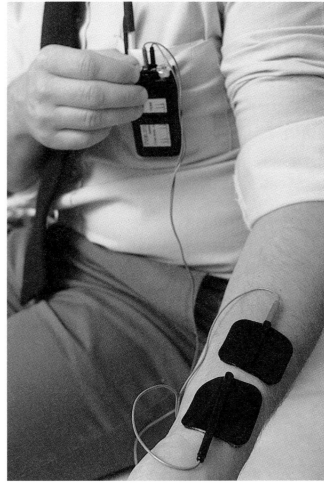

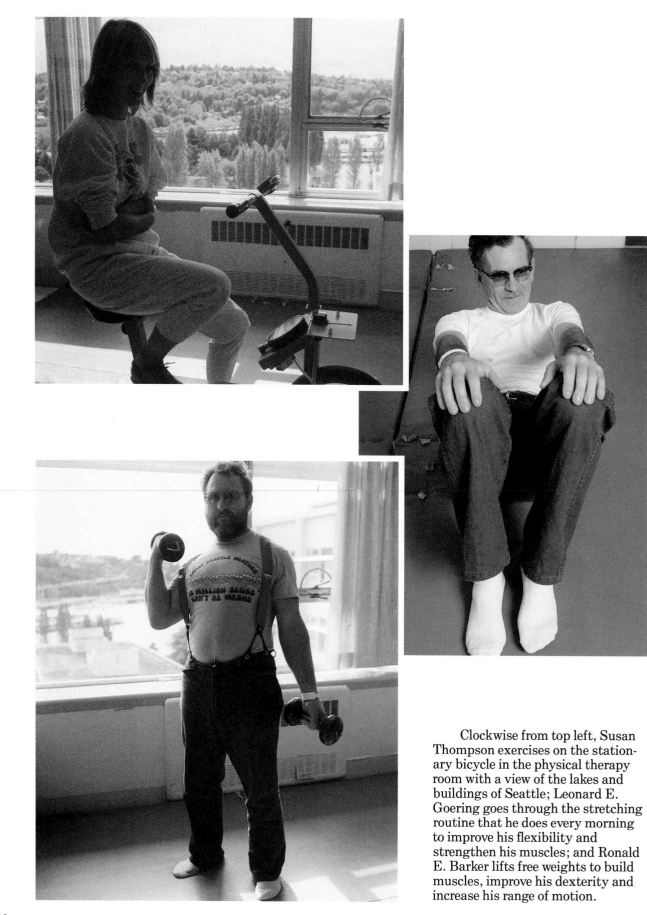

Clockwise from top left, Susan Thompson exercises on the stationary bicycle in the physical therapy room with a view of the lakes and buildings of Seattle; Leonard E. Goering goes through the stretching routine that he does every morning to improve his flexibility and strengthen his muscles; and Ronald E. Barker lifts free weights to build muscles, improve his dexterity and increase his range of motion.

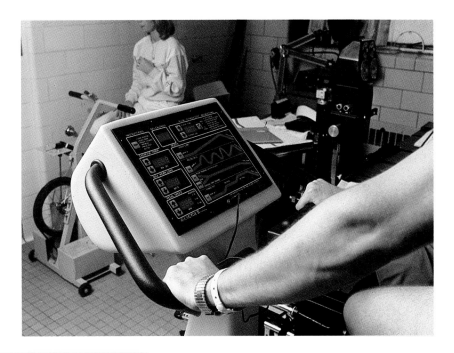

Steve Elliott works out on a computerized exercise cycle that tells him his pulse, aerobic workload and pedal speed. Exercise is an important part of the clinic program because it strengthens the body and helps the person regain strength and endurance in long-neglected muscles.

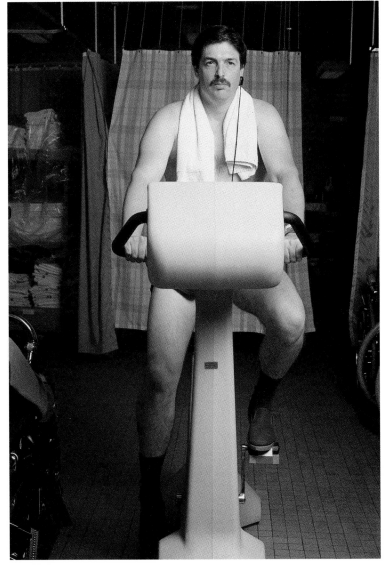

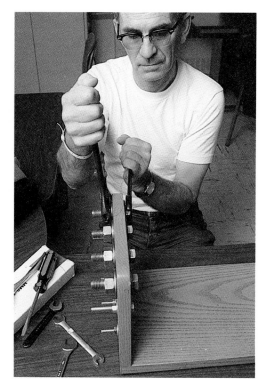

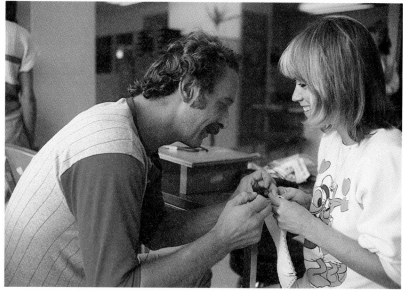

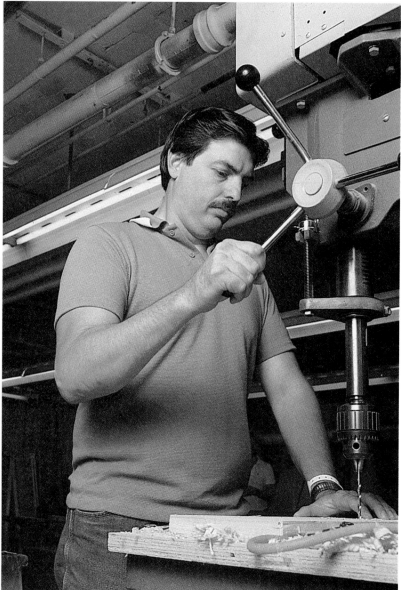

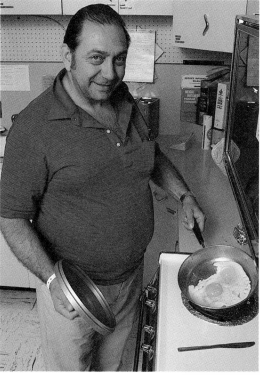

Occupational and vocational therapy are used at the clinic to help people realize just what they are capable of doing. Many pain patients who have been inactive for a long time are surprised at their abilities. On the opposite page, clockwise from far left, Leonard E. Goering works with nuts and bolts to improve his dexterity; Clifford G. Dennis, Jr., and Susan Thompson craft leather pouches in an exercise designed to show them they can be active for an hour or so without giving in to their pain; and Steve Elliot, a carpenter, learns less painful ways to use the tools of his trade. On this page, above, Dick Calderon shows off perfectly fried eggs in the kitchen that allows patients to learn how to function well around the home; at right, Susan Thompson rides in a mockup of an automobile to learn how to sit in a car with a minimum amount of pain—something she couldn't do previously.

12

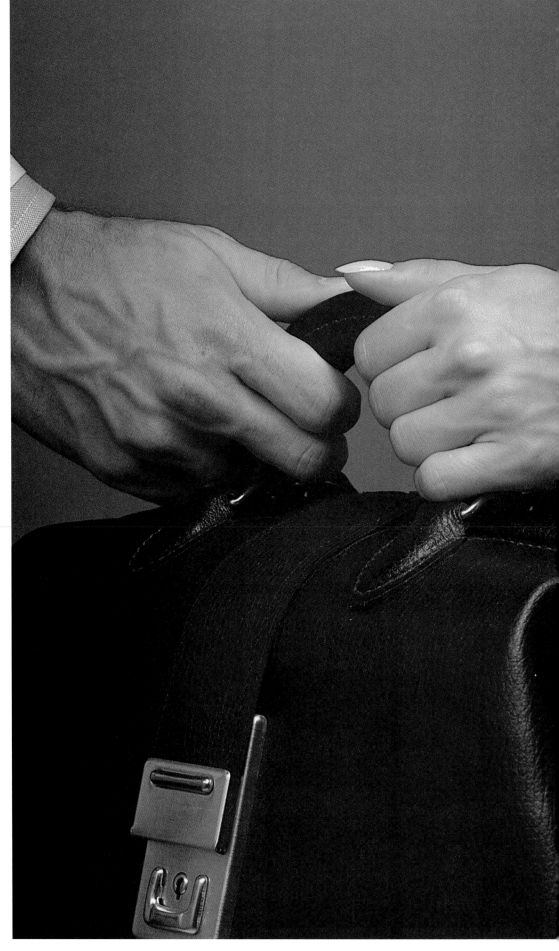

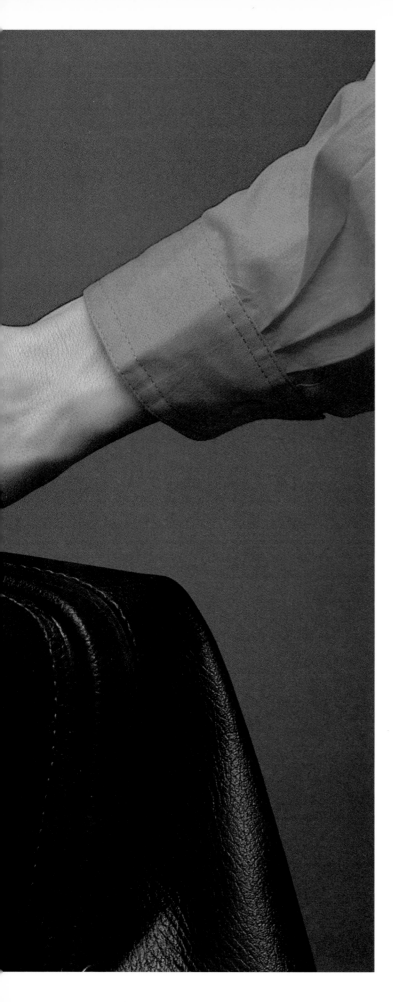

Working with the Medical System

It's a buyer's market out there. Smarten up and become an educated medical consumer.

Glut.

If there's one word that describes the medical professional today, that's it. Everywhere you turn, there's a doctor, alternative practitioner, hospital or pharmaceutical company chasing after you.

Your pain is their profit.

Glut.

The Department of Health, Education and Welfare predicted there will be more than 600,000 doctors in America by the year 1990. They said that's anywhere from 5,000 to 50,000 more than we need, and that's just the overall picture. Doctors have always flocked to the big cities, making the glut in urban areas even worse.

Glut.

Hospitals have become so desperate for the $ick and injured that they market themselves like mouthwash. Newspaper, radio and television ads bark their come-ons. A Las Vegas hospital once gave discounts and discount lottery tickets to lure customers. Some hospitals in Los Angeles are rumored to have offered luxury cars and paid vacations to doctors who referred a lot of patients. The latest trend has hospitals offering money-back-guaranteed get-well service, an unprecedented development in medical care.

Why all the hard sell? Too many empty rooms. There are now at least 7,000 hospitals in America—about 1,500 more than we need, say industry analysts. They predict that hospital closings may be the wave of the future.

Glut.

Drugs, both prescription and over-the-counter, are a multibillion-dollar business. The *Physicians' Desk Reference*, the reference book of the drug industry, devotes an entire, tiny-print index page to painkillers, listing more than 250 different types. Seems like everyone is trying to make a killing in painkillers.

Despite the ominous tones, this abundance actually is good news for you. The glut translates into a buyer's market for medical care. You can now shop comparatively for the best doctor, hospital and drug at the most economical price. All you need is a little knowledge about how to become a smart medical consumer. In this chapter, we'll give you pointers.

PICKING A WINNER

People in pain usually surrender themselves to a physician, trusting that his or her skills will relieve the agony. But did you ever consider that it may be *your* skill at choosing the right physician that holds the key to pain relief?

As in any profession, doctors can be good, bad or mediocre. Since chronic pain is often one of the most difficult conditions to diagnose and treat, the ability, attitude and determination of your doctor is vital.

How do you pick a winner when it comes to doctors? Here are some tips.

First of all, make sure your kindly physician is actually a doctor! Don't smirk. A study by a congressional committee reported that more than 10,000 bogus medical certificates have been issued to practicing phonies. Some of the "doctors" don't even have high school degrees, much less M.D.'s.

If you have doubts about your doctor, the American Medical Association (AMA) suggests that you visit your library and consult two books, the *Directory of Medical Specialists*, and the *American Medical Directory*. If you can't locate the name of your doctor in these, contact the officials at your state medical licensing agency and ask them to check. If they come up empty, you may have uncovered a fraud. Steer clear.

FINDING DR. GOOD-STETHOSCOPE

But just being licensed isn't enough. Dr. Nelson Hendler of Johns Hopkins Hospital feels people in pain need doctors with specific qualities.

"You should look for a physician who will take the time to listen to your problem, someone genuine, warm, empathetic and sincere. You need an hour, an hour and a half to take a good history. Someone who gets you in and out in 10 minutes is not hearing the whole story.

"You need a doctor who is willing to refer you to other physicians. No one doctor knows everything about pain. And just as important, you must find a doctor who will be aware of the psychological impact pain has had on your life—things like depression, sleeplessness, marital problems and financial difficulties. Your physician should try to assist you with these areas, not try to blame your pain on them. They are the result of your pain, not the cause," says Dr. Hendler.

To find a doctor with these qualities, according to Dr. Hendler, you should ask friends, neighbors and business associates for recommendations. Then book an appointment and judge for yourself.

A study by researchers at the University of New Mexico School of Medicine offers another view on what makes a good doctor. The researchers observed interactions between doctors and their patients and then asked the patients what attributes they preferred. The most recurrent responses were: a friendly greeting; a preview of what might happen to them next; a willingness to listen to them; and general thoughtfulness.

Warren Bosley, M.D., a pediatrician in Grand Island, Nebraska, says you can quickly gauge a doctor's thoughtfulness by studying his or her waiting room.

"You will want to walk into an attractive office where you are greeted by people who are pleased to see you," Dr. Bosley says. "You should find an office arrangement that permits the receptionist, secretary or doctor to interview you in a private setting, where your answers to their questions are not heard by everyone."

Most doctors, medical organizations and consumer groups feel that once you have privacy, you and your doctor should have clear and open communication. That means you should be free to ask questions, not just take orders.

"Your doctor should be willing to speak openly and patiently with you," advises Charles B. Inlander, executive director of the People's Medical Society (PMS), a medical care watchdog group for consumers. "Don't forget, however, that it takes two to communicate. You will need to ask questions."

"Doctors aren't mind readers," reminds Frederic C. McDuffie, M.D., senior vice president of medical affairs for the Arthritis Foundation. "It's in your best interest to be specific about how you feel and what you think. Don't feel stupid if you have to ask the same question again. Part of a doctor's job is also to be an educator."

The questions you should ask, according to the People's Medical Society, include:

- To what hospital does the doctor admit patients?
- What arrangements are there for stand-in doctors when your doctor is not available?
- Will the doctor prescribe generic drugs?
- What will the treatment cost, and will the doctor accept direct payments from Medicare or an insurance company?

BAD PRACTICES

As director of the Mensana Clinic, Dr. Hendler often sees chronic pain patients who have previously had less than sympathetic care. From studying their cases, he's noticed warning signals that may help you quickly spot doctors who might not be suited for your particular problem.

"First and foremost, if the doctor says it's all in your head, or you are imagining the pain, he's not the doctor to help you. If the doctor says 'It can't hurt that much,' or 'I operated on you, you should be better now,' or 'How can you still hurt?' consider finding a new doctor.

"Watch out for doctors who

Become Your Own Expert

When it comes to your pain, one doctor will give you only one point of view. That's why *you* should get informed—to find out about *other* approaches to treating your pain.

Fortunately, becoming your own expert isn't as hard as you might think. Start by calling your public library. Its reference librarian can tell you about other community resources, including recorded explanations of medical topics that are available free by phone in many places. If that's not enough, try the local hospital—most have public information or education departments that can answer your questions. Many also have medical libraries where the staff can show you which medical books or journals to use. It's a good idea to ask for a medical dictionary, too, so you can wade through complicated medical jargon.

You gain expertise by asking good questions, so always ask about the full range of treatments available; how successful they're likely to be; what risks are involved; and what will happen if you don't do anything at all.

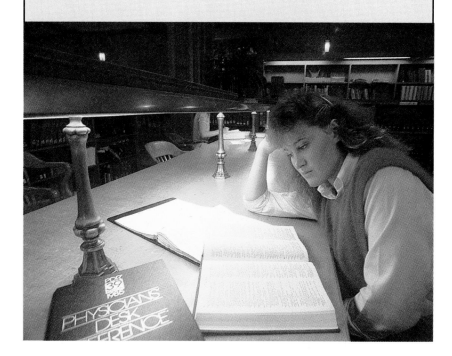

blame you for the pain just because they can't explain it," continues Dr. Hendler. "If your doctor couples this with being unwilling or afraid to refer you to another doctor, I'd be concerned.

"There are also some specific pain buzz words to be aware of. If your doctor mentions 'hysterical pain,' 'conversion reaction pain,' 'imaginary pain,' 'psychosomatic or psychogenic pain,' get out of the office as quickly as possible. These are all fancy ways of saying the pain is in your head," Dr. Hendler warns.

DRESS FOR SUCCESS

Now that we've seen the speck in some doctors' eyes, let's not lose sight of the log in our own. Are you a good patient, or is your doctor indifferent and less effective because you stink—figuratively and literally? (As you'll find out in a second, this is less outrageous than it sounds.)

David Klein, Ph.D., of Michigan State University, a former social science professor, decided to find out. In a detailed study, he polled doctors on what medical conditions and social characteristics they disliked in patients. Heading the list was mental illness, mentioned by 56.7 percent of the doctors in the study. That characteristic was followed by alcoholism (55.8 percent), "dirty, smelly, poor hygiene," (44.9 percent), drug addiction (42.1 percent) and obesity (33.5 percent).

"Because they themselves are very self-disciplined, doctors tend to feel that any patient who lacks self-discipline and is willing to indulge himself is a bad patient culpable for his own condition," says Dr. Klein.

Another study confirms that you should "dress for medical success." Behavioral scientists at the University of New Mexico have found that the best-dressed patients received better care and more attention than their shabby counterparts.

These findings suggest that neat clothing, along with routine social etiquette and good personal hygiene, may get you better care and treatment.

GETTING DOWN TO BUSINESS

Now that you've cleaned up your act, you should be mentally prepared to help your doctor by giving him as much information as possible.

"The most effective way you can take part in this discussion is to prepare in advance," says Linda Hughey Holt, M.D., author of *The American Medical Association Guide to Woman Care*. "You'd be surprised at the things you'll forget when you're in the doctor's office. Among the items to list are your symptoms—all of them—and how long and how often you've had them; all medications you take, either regularly or frequently, including oral contraceptives, aspirin, sleeping pills, vitamins, laxatives and tranquilizers. List your allergies, particularly allergies to drugs such as penicillin. Take along your immunization record, if possible."

Dr. Holt and the AMA say that other things to note include:

- A history of your general health, including major illnesses, surgery,

---

Say What, Doc?

"Is your chronic but idiopathic pain referred, systemic or merely psychogenic?" Say what, doc? Sometimes physicians use 25-cent words when a nickel or a penny would do. Use this list to make their mumbo-jumbo painfully clear:

Analgesic—painkiller.

Acute pain—sharp, short-term pain, usually after injuries.

Chronic pain—pain that persists for a long time.

Contusion—a bruise.

Dermatitis—a catch-all phrase for any inflammation of the skin.

Edema—swelling.

Idiopathic—of unknown cause.

Neuralgia—a sharp, spasmlike pain recurring at intervals, usually caused by nerve damage.

Psychogenic—resulting from mental or emotional causes.

Referred pain—pain felt in one area of the body due to disease or injury somewhere else.

Rheumatalgia—chronic pain from rheumatism.

Subclinical—having no visible symptoms.

Systemic—affecting the whole body.

Sheila Cross, M.D.
Albany, N.Y.
The "Doctor Shuffle"

When a routine knee injury mushroomed into a tormenting battle against relentless pain, Sheila Cross, M.D., discovered that her medical degree could not shield her from a demoralizing medical nightmare—the "what pain?" doctor shuffle. Two years, 12 doctors, 5 operations, a lost practice and $100,000 in bills later, she finally found relief. But it was a long, hard road.

"They said I had 'hysterical' pain, then low pain tolerance, then that I had the pain because my marriage was bad, which was totally untrue," says Dr. Cross. "They said I was dependent on drugs and invented the pain to stay on drugs. After that they decided I was crazy and wanted to ship me to the psychiatric ward."

What Dr. Cross really had was sympathetic dystrophy and an entrapped nerve above her knee that resulted in constant, searing pain 3 inches below the knee.

When her original orthopedic surgeon and physical therapist failed in their attempts to ease the pain, she was passed to a neurologist. The nerve man decreed "depression" as the cause and gave her mood-lifting drugs.

"The pain grew worse. An orthopedic surgeon performed some pain blocks using drugs to deaden certain areas. It didn't work," she says.

A neurosurgeon came next. He told her to tough it out like a man would. She got another neurosurgeon. He told her to wait it out. She waited. Eleven agonizing weeks later neurosurgeon number 2 decided to operate. He found swollen, abnormal nerves in the lower knee area. He severed them, sealed them off and pronounced Dr. Cross pain free. She wasn't. He told her to see a psychiatrist. She relented. The psychiatrist said her

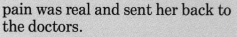

pain was real and sent her back to the doctors.

The parade continued. Another neurologist, back to her original orthopedic surgeon, then to an anesthesiologist for 5 more painful blocks. Back to neurosurgeon number 2 for another operation—and, finally, relief for at least some of her pain. She went to a new neurologist in Syracuse, New York, hoping to find total relief, then to a second psychiatrist. She was at the end of her rope.

"Finally, I heard about the innovative pain research at the Mensana Clinic outside Baltimore, Maryland. I went. A team of specialists there assured me my pain was very real. I have sympathetic dystrophy and they promised to correct it.

"Within 24 hours I had a diagnosis, a treatment plan and the promise of an effective cure."

Dr. Sheila Cross had finally found the right doctors.

When to See a Doctor for Pain

Pain Site	See a Doctor for:	Get Emergency Treatment for:
Abdomen	Cramps, accompanied by nausea, fever, vomiting, or diarrhea, if symptoms last 2 to 3 days. Sharp pain in the upper right side below the ribs; may be accompanied by fever. Occasional bouts of pain in the center or upper abdomen that is relieved by vomiting. Burning pain on one side only; skin is tender along site of pain. Pain in the lower abdomen accompanied by bouts of diarrhea; may be accompanied by fever Painful menstrual periods and heavy or smelly vaginal discharge between periods; may be accompanied by fever.	Cramps, accompanied by nausea, fever, vomiting or diarrhea, along with extreme weakness. Any severe pain lasting more than 1 hour that's not relieved by vomiting, accompanied by fever or severe constipation. Severe pain in the lower abdomen in early pregnancy.
Back	Pain in the small of the back on one side just above the waist, which moves to the groin; may be accompanied by fever.	Pain that comes on suddenly following an injury to the back, accompanied by loss of bladder or bowel control, difficulty moving any limb or numbness or tingling in any limb.
Bones		Severe pain or misshapen limb following an injury.
Chest	In women, pain accompanied by one or more lumps in the breasts.	Sudden pain, discomfort or tightening that lasts more than 5 to 15 minutes and/or radiates from the center of the chest to the jaw, neck or arms. Pain extending down the arm to the wrist that stops after 5 minutes of rest. Radiating pain in the chest, shortness of breath or pain that is worse when you inhale.
Ears	Pain in one or both ears, especially when accompanied by a discharge.	
Eyes	Pain in one or both eyes.	Pain in one or both eyes, accompanied by redness or blurred or impaired vision.
Genitals	Painful or frequent urination, discharge, itchiness, redness, swelling, lumps, sores or painful intercourse. In men, pain and swelling in one or both testes.	
Head/Face	Red rash, dry cough, sore eyes, running nose, and/ or swelling at the base of the skull or at the sides of the neck. Severe throbbing in the temples, a feeling of malaise and the scalp is sensitive to touch. Recurrent headaches that are present on waking and accompanied by nausea or vomiting.	Sudden neck pain accompanied by severe headache, pain on bending the head forward, nausea and vomiting, sensitivity to light, drowsiness or confusion.
Joints	Pain in the elbow, wrist or hand that occurs only when the joint is bent a certain way, if the pain persists or worsens after a few days.	Pain in any joint accompanied by redness and fever.
Legs/Ankles Feet/Toes	Painful knee that sometimes sticks or gives way.	Painful, swollen, tender calf that may be accompanied by a red cordlike swelling of a vein.
Mouth/Tongue	Pain all over the tongue. Painful, red and swollen gums accompanied by bad breath or foul taste in the mouth.	
Neck/Throat	Swelling and tenderness of the neck accompanied by painful swallowing and fever lasting more than 48 hours. Stiff neck that has gotten worse for several months, accompanied by tingling or numbness in the arm or hand, especially if you are over age 50.	Sudden neck pain that may be accompanied by severe headache, nausea and vomiting, sensitivity to bright light, drowsiness or confusion. Sudden pain after a jolt to the neck, accompanied by difficulty in controlling arm or leg muscles.

hospitalizations or injuries and your health in childhood.

- Health problems of close relatives, living or dead, including anemia, allergies, arthritis, abnormal bleeding, cancer, diabetes, endocrine diseases, epilepsy, gout, heart disease, high blood pressure, jaundice, kidney disease, mental retardation, migraines, obesity, psychiatric illness and tuberculosis.
- Specific problems you may have, such as breathing problems, coughs, bleeding, digestive trouble, insomnia, menstrual problems.
- Specific details about your lifestyle: your job, living situation, activities, personal habits and sex life. (The doctor is not prying; these are vital factors in your overall health picture and can be a key to analyzing your symptoms.)

GETTING HELP

Numerous reference books, organizations and special services are available to help you decide on a doctor, better understand the one you have or get a second opinion, or offer tips on how to make the doctor/patient relationship better. Your local librarian may be able to help you with the books, including the *Directory of Medical Specialists* and the *American Medical Directory*. Other helpful sources include:

- The People's Medical Society. This is a national, nonprofit organization formed to give information to private citizens and to push for reforms in the medical system. Annual membership is $15. For information on joining, write to The People's Medical Society, 14 East Minor Street, Emmaus, PA 18049.
- The Second Surgical Opinion Program Hotline (1-800-638-6833; in Maryland, 1-800-492-6603). This group will locate a board-certified physician in your area who will give a second opinion on suggested nonemer-

gency surgery. There is no charge for their services.

- The American Academy of Family Physicians. For a list of certified family physicians in your area, send a stamped, self-addressed envelope to 1740 West 92nd Street, Kansas City, MO 64114.

HOSPITABLE HOSPITALS

How would you like to spend a wonderful week at Club Hospital, a thrilling vacation paradise? We offer a stiff bed in a colorless room that you will share with an infectious, wheezing stranger. We'll plunge needles into your body every chance we get, either to squish some unidentified chemical in or to painfully drag something out.

You'll get three beyond-bland meals a day, brought right to your bed by a team of surly, overworked, underpaid nurses. We'll force-feed you sleeping pills and keep you confined to your bed for almost the entire week.

If you're good, we may even let you see your doctor for, say, a minute every day or so.

Best of all, you get all this for a mere $500 a day, not including expenses.

Talk about pain! How many of you would sign up for a vacation like that? Yet many people go to hospitals for the same reason they take vacations—to recover from the end-stage pains of overwork, exhaustion, illness and stress, and to gain physical rejuvenation. Granted, a hospital stay will never rival a Caribbean vacation, but there are ways to make your stay more pleasant.

FINDING A HOSPITAL

How do you find a hospitable hospital or pain center?

"You ask any doctor you know, 'Where do you go when *you* are sick? Where do you send your children? Who is your surgeon?'" advises Dr. Hendler.

"If your problem is chronic pain, you must choose a multidisciplinary

Have a Painless Hospital Stay

Face it, the hospital's not the best place for comfort. Just when you've tuned out the noise, an army of nurses stick thermometers in your mouth and needles in your arm. But there's a lot you can do to keep the painful pokes and jabs to a minimum, says Jack Weinberger, R.N., a critical-care nurse in Seattle.

"Communicate with the people who are hurting you," he stresses. Instead of enduring frequent blood tests, ask to have lab work consolidated so all the jabbing is done at once. If you don't want to be disturbed, say so. Above all, refuse any procedure you don't understand. And when pain is unavoidable, never hold your breath. Instead, take deep breaths and exhale slowly. It will hurt less.

center where you will be seen by a lot of doctors. The cornerstone of treating pain is making a proper diagnosis. No one physician can do that without the assistance of others." (See chapter 11.)

Two other qualities to seek (or demand) in a good hospital are patient representatives and an infection-control physician. Some hospitals have them; many don't.

A patient representative (also called a patient advocate or ombudsman) is a troubleshooter employed by the hospital solely to serve the patient by taking care of any problems that might arise. Their power and exact functions vary from hospital to hospital, but the trend is to give them more and more authority to help them effectively solve patient problems.

Chronic pain patients, whose hospitalization may be lengthy and laden with tests, are particularly likely to benefit from the services of a patient representative, according to Alexandra Gekas, director of the National Society of Patient Representatives of the American Hospital Association.

"Anytime patients or their families have questions and don't know where to go, become unhappy or frustrated, or have any problem that doesn't fall into the routine areas of responsibility, they can call the patient representative," Ms. Gekas says.

"We will do almost anything, from getting more information about your illness, to getting the appropriate health professional to explain an upcoming procedure more clearly, to changing your room if that's necessary, or even bringing your doctor back so he can alleviate your fears."

Ms. Gekas says 52 percent of all hospitals in America now have a patient representative. The way to find out if your hospital has one is simple: Call the switchboard and ask.

"Make sure you are clear about what you want," Ms. Gekas advises. "Switchboard operators often confuse the patient representative for a service representative, the person who deals with insurance coverage. Be specific. Get the patient representative on the phone if you can. Ask them what they think of the hospital,

what their function is, and how much authority they wield."

GETTING WORSE, NOT BETTER

You're in the hospital to get rid of pain, not add to it. Yet a major study by doctors and researchers at the Centers for Disease Control in Atlanta came to the shocking conclusion that an estimated four million hospital and nursing home patients per year *acquire* hospital-bred infections during their stay.

The good news is that some hospitals are concerned enough about this trend to establish an infection surveillance and control program. The Centers for Disease Control say such programs work. In a parallel study, they found that hospitals employing measures including an infection-control physician, along with one infection-control nurse per 250 beds, were able to reduce the infection rate by 32 percent. Hospitals without the infection-control program had an infection rate that increased 18 percent over six years.

That is a whopping 50 percent difference. While you have the hospital switchboard operator on the phone to ask about the patient representative, also ask about the infection-control program. If the hospital has both, you're in business.

QUESTIONS BRING ANSWERS FOR YOUR PAIN

Don't let your questioning end there. The People's Medical Society says that before you trade your street duds for a rearless hospital gown, you should blister the admissions officer's ears with a flurry of questions, including:

- How much will it cost? (All of it, including doctors' fees, hospital costs and extras.) Will they accept your insurance? Once you have a figure, shop around for the best hospital at the best price.
- How's the food? Check out the kitchen. Ask the hospital dietitian. Sample it. If it's bad and you still must go to that hospital,

consider bringing your own food, or having visitors drop off balanced, nutritious meals. (This is only for patients who aren't on a special diet.) If you take this step, make sure you don't end up paying for hospital food you never ate.

- Is the hospital licensed by the state? Accredited by the Joint Commission on the Accreditation of Hospitals? Is the administrator licensed by, or a member of, the American College of Hospital Administrators? The answers should be yes.
- How many nurses are on staff? Look for a patient-to-nurse ratio no greater than four to one (two to one in intensive care). What's the ratio of registered nurses (R.N.) to licensed practical nurses (L.P.N.)? Registered nurses have more training, up to four years of college and sometimes even master's degrees, while L.P.N.'s can have as little as one year of nursing school.
- What is the secondary infection rate among surgical patients?
- How many surgical procedures of the type you require does the hospital perform each year?

The PMS also suggests taking a walking tour of the hospital. Are the floors clean? How does the place smell? Note the personal hygiene of the doctors and nurses. Are the uniforms of the housekeepers, orderlies and security guards clean? Are the rooms clean and well kept?

And finally, ask yourself, your doctor and your second-opinion doctors, "Do I really need to be in the hospital? If so, how soon can I get out?"

An excellent reference book is *Take This Book to the Hospital with You*, by Charles B. Inlander, Executive Director, People's Medical Society, and Ed Weiner. Contact PMS at the address given on page 157 for information on ordering the book.

CHOOSING THE RIGHT PAIN RELIEVER

For the treatment of pain, doctors and hospitals usually go hand-in-

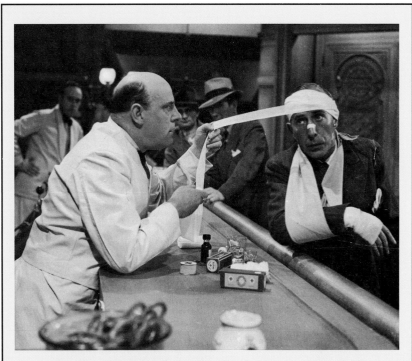

Pain Relief? I'll Drink to That!

Those Dodge City docs weren't all wrong—alcohol can be an effective pain reliever, if used properly. According to Tom Ferguson, M.D., editor of *Medical Self Care* magazine, it's "as effective as aspirin for most people" and is especially useful in emergency situations with short-term acute pain or occasionally for arthritis pain. But don't routinely use alcohol for pain relief—alcohol is addictive, and some people can't handle it. "If you don't have a problem with alcohol, 1 or 2 drinks can be quite useful," says Dr. Ferguson, but drinking more than that can harm your health. And never mix alcohol and painkilling drugs—the combination can be deadly.

hand with one other useful treatment: drugs. And getting the best medicine you can find is very important.

Choosing a painkilling (analgesic) drug is like choosing any other tool. First, consider the job at hand. Do you have a headache? A toothache? Menstrual cramps? Back strain? Achy joints? Some analgesics work well for certain forms of pain but not so well—or not at all—for others. The

159

painkilling tool you choose depends partly on the task.

The *size* of the job also dictates the type of painkiller you need. Heavy-duty pain—broken bones, postsurgical healing, an extracted wisdom tooth—call for industrial-strength painkilling tools such as morphine or Demerol, which are only available by prescription.

But no matter what type of pain reliever you use, you can get the most relief from as little medicine as possible if you learn something about how they work and also ask your doctor or pharmacist the right questions.

To start off, let's learn about do-it-yourself pain relievers—the kind you can find on the drugstore shelf.

WHAT YOU SHOULD KNOW ABOUT OVER-THE-COUNTER PAIN MEDICINE

"Take two acetylsalicylic acid and call me in the morning."

That chemical name might not ring a bell, but the phrase is so familiar, such a part of healing lore and practice, that you know what we're talking about: aspirin.

Anyone who's ever suffered a splitting headache, back strain or other moderate body moan probably thinks of aspirin when they think of pain relief. Aspirin also goes by the trade names Bayer, Empirin and Bufferin, among others, and it reduces fever and inflammation as well as pain. Aspirin probably dampens pain by controlling the production of prostaglandins, hormonelike substances made from essential fatty acids that are produced by most of the body's cells. Prostaglandins are necessary for cells to function properly, but sometimes cells produce too many and, for some unknown reason, that generates pain.

Although aspirin may be the best known and most time-tested moderate pain reliever, it's certainly not the only one. Acetaminophen is a relative newcomer to the painkilling scene. Datril, Tylenol and other brand-name versions of this analgesic relieve pain but not inflammation.

A third pain reliever in this class, ibuprofen, goes by names such as Nuprin and Advil. Like aspirin, ibuprofen controls the production of pain-triggering prostaglandins. But ibuprofen appears to be a stronger pain reliever than aspirin. One 200-milligram tablet of ibuprofen is as effective as two 325-milligram tablets of aspirin.

Of the three, which is best?

That depends on what ails you. Both aspirin and acetaminophen work equally well to reduce pain and fever, but only aspirin reduces inflammation. So of the two, aspirin is better for arthritis or a sprained ankle. Aspirin also works better for menstrual cramps than acetaminophen because it affects the action of cramp-producing prostaglandins. That's if the cramps are fairly mild. But if they're pretty strong—the kind that make you want to drop everything and curl up with a heating pad—ibuprofen is effective and relatively safe. And because ibuprofen gives more power for the punch than aspirin, it may be just the right tool for people with arthritis or other chronic conditions that require lots of pain relief.

None of these drugs is free of potential side effects. So your choice will also depend on how well you tolerate various types. Some people who take aspirin experience stomach upset or gastrointestinal bleeding, especially if they take it regularly (four or more days a week) or in large doses (more than 15 tablets a week). For them, acetaminophen—which doesn't upset the stomach—may be the better of the two.

No matter which pain reliever you choose, always read the label—*every word.* The manufacturers tell you how much to take, how often and when, and who should avoid the drug entirely or consult their doctor before taking it. Each of these drugs has a list of medical conditions that also could prevent their use.

Few people intend to hurt themselves with aspirin or other analgesics. But if you have arthritis, chronic back pain or other types of persistent, nagging pain, you could find yourself taking quite a few pills to get through the day—or night—comfortably. And the fact that these useful painkilling tools are so easily available can lull

Marge Knowlton
Stillwater, Minn.
Addiction to Painkillers

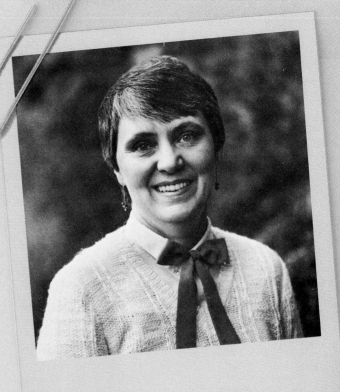

Marge Knowlton's "drug problem" started in high school, but it was perfectly legit.

She had a long history of skull-splitting tension headaches—the kind that begin in the neck and shoulders and creep to the head. And all too often, Marge's headaches lasted not for hours but for *days*.

Aspirin was powerless against these monster headaches. So Marge's doctor prescribed Darvon and Valium.

"The prescription drugs killed the pain, but they also made me feel good," says Marge. "I remember getting a headache, taking my pills and going to work as a cashier at the supermarket. I felt real spacey, but I *liked* the feeling—so much, in fact, that I began to actually look forward to getting the headaches so I could take the drugs."

Eventually, the drugs began to mess up Marge's life. Married, with two school-age children, she could barely drag herself through the day. She had to force herself to shower and dress by the time the children got home from school at 3:15.

"Getting dinner on the table was a major chore," Marge recalls. "My husband knew something was wrong but didn't know what to do. And I thought I was just plain going crazy."

The turning point came when Marge mentioned her vegetative condition to a former counselor, who commented, "Sounds like chemical dependency to me."

He was right. Marge went to her family doctor, who recommended withdrawal from the drugs. Marge knew she was hooked pretty badly, so she entered treatment for drug addiction at a private rehabilitation center.

"An addiction is the same whether you're hooked on alcohol or medicine, legal drugs or illegal drugs," says Marge. "So the treatment worked for me. I still go to a support group. The spirituality helps tremendously."

Marge still gets headaches, but they're less frequent and not nearly as painful. To relieve the pain, Marge takes aspirin and applies a heating pad to her neck. If she feels a headache coming on, she wards off pain by meditating or listening to relaxation tapes. When she feels stressed, Marge practices progressive muscle relaxation to reduce tension, the root cause of her headaches.

With these tools, Marge is now able to live without the dangerous chemicals that she had become dependent on to dull her pain.

Why Not Heroin?

Many people, desperate to find relief from cancer pain for themselves or loved ones, wonder why heroin isn't used in the U.S. to kill pain.

"Heroin is no more effective for pain than morphine," says William Beaver, M.D., a professor of pharmacology at Georgetown University, Washington, D.C.

Why is it, then, that some cancer patients still don't get relief with morphine or other narcotics? "Many doctors don't use them to their fullest potential," says Dr. Beaver. So make sure you or your loved one gets the right drugs in the right amounts.

the most savvy consumer into a false sense of security. And, as it turns out, the biggest risk of taking non-prescription pain relievers is accidental overdose. Remember that it's just like the ads say: These drugs are safe and effective *when used as directed.*

You could also direct yourself to a copy of the *Physicians' Desk Reference for Nonprescription Drugs.* It's an excellent source of information about using over-the-counter pain relievers. Your local library probably has a copy. If not, your pharmacist may.

A SAFER WAY TO TAKE ASPIRIN

Say that, for one reason or another, you choose aspirin for your pain. You can lessen its effect on your digestive tract by drinking 8 ounces of a nonalcoholic beverage with your pills. That will help the aspirin dissolve more quickly and be absorbed faster. (If taken with alcohol, aspirin is more irritating.)

Or try enteric-coated aspirin. *Enteric* refers to the small intestine—the place where this type of aspirin dissolves, 6 hours after you swallow it. Needless to say, it's easier on your stomach than regular aspirin. Also needless to say, it takes longer to work.

THE NARCOTICS SQUAD

You have an impacted wisdom tooth pulled. Or you ski into a tree and dislocate a shoulder. Or your arthritis is so bad you can hardly walk. Aspirin or aspirin alternatives will hardly fill the bill: They work at the site of the pain, reducing the number of pain messages received by the nerve endings in the skin, muscles, joints, ligaments or gums. These drugs have very little effect on your brain, which ultimately registers all pain. For moderate to severe pain, your doctor may prescribe a narcotic pain reliever: either codeine, propoxyphene (Darvon), meperidine (Demerol) or oxycodone (Percodan). Narcotic painkillers will relieve all but the most excruciating pain. Narcotics work by masking the way your brain registers pain signals.

Sounds great, you say. Can I buy these over the counter, like aspirin?

No, for two reasons: They're addictive, which means your mind and body habituate to them. Moreover, your tolerance builds, thus requiring larger and larger doses to do the job.

"All these drugs have a potential for addiction to some degree, especially if taken in slightly larger doses or for slightly longer than recommended," explains Charles Green, a registered pharmacist in Stockton, California.

And narcotics can spell big trouble if you take them along with any other drugs that slow down the brain or cental nervous system, such as diazepam (Valium).

"If someone is taking Percodan, for example, and then begins to take Valium, he or she may react so severely that they end up in the emergency room," says Green.

Green sums up the proper role of narcotics this way: "Narcotics are useful for a given period of time only. You need to take care of the cause. The sooner you can wean yourself off the medicine, the healthier you will be."

But what if you *do* need a narcotic for a "given period of time"? Which of these heavy-duty pain relievers will your doctor prescribe for you? That depends on two factors: How badly do you hurt? How long is the pain likely to last?

"Codeine and Darvon are fairly similar in the way they relieve pain," says Green. "The major benefit is that they're more powerful than aspirin or its substitutes. And when taken properly, they can be taken for a longer time than Demerol or Percodan without leading to addiction."

The drawbacks?

"Codeine may cause constipation or nausea," says Green. "And you can build up a tolerance."

So doctors usually prescribe codeine or Darvon for long-term or moderate pain. Percodan and Demerol, as well as Dilaudid, morphine, methadone and Levodromoran, are all excellent for short-term or severe pain, such as that resulting from dental surgery, an injury or outpatient surgery. The drawbacks are that they may cause nausea or light-headedness and they are *very* addicting. Plus, they can turn you into a zombie, leaving you apathetic, unable to remember clearly or make sound judgments. So, unless you were severely ill, you wouldn't want to rely on either Demerol or Percodan for much more than a week or so if a less powerful painkiller would do the job.

You can avoid taking more narcotics than you need by working closely with your doctor and pharmacist, points out Green.

"Say you hurt your arm on the job. Your doctor gives you a few Percodans. A week later, you feel you need a refill. Fine. Then you may feel you need more pills because you still have a painful twinge or so. At that point, the doctor shouldn't refill the prescription without making an appointment with you to find out *why* you're still in pain. Is the arm infected? What's going on?

"You may still need pain relief, but something less powerful than a narcotic may be enough. Perhaps acetaminophen would do the job," explains Green.

"It's fairly common practice for doctors to start people taking a drug such as Percodan, then step down to codeine and end with acetaminophen or another over-the-counter analgesic," says Green. "Or your doctor may start to treat pain with 1 grain (a pharmaceutical measurement) of codeine, work down to ½ grain, then ¼ grain. That's one method to reduce risk of addiction to pain-relieving drugs."

MUSCLE RELAXANTS FOR STRAINS AND SPRAINS

Strains, sprains, spasms and other muscle injuries often call for a slightly different approach to pain relief: compounds that relax taut muscles, taking the bite out of pain in nearby nerve endings. Muscle relaxant drugs include diazepam (Valium), methocarbamol (Robaxin), and orphenadrine (Disipal, Estamul, Norflex).

Each muscle relaxant has its own set of possible side effects, but all tend to make you drowsy or light-headed, at least when you first take them. So above all, don't operate a car or dangerous machinery until you know how this drug is going to affect you. And, unless your doctor tells you otherwise, don't take a muscle relaxant with anything else that slows you down, such as alcohol, barbiturates or other narcotic drugs for pain. In fact, it's a good idea to tell your doctor about any other prescription or nonprescription drugs you take if he or she prescribes muscle relaxants. That includes antihistamines or other medicine for hay fever, allergies or colds; sedatives, tranquilizers or other medicine to help you sleep; medicine for seizures or depression; or MAO (monoamine oxidase) inhibitors. All those drugs can increase the odds or severity of an unhealthy reaction to muscle relaxants.

QUESTIONS TO ASK YOUR DOCTOR ABOUT PRESCRIPTION DRUGS

To get the most relief with the least trouble from prescription pain relievers, ask your doctor or pharmacist the following questions:

- What kind of medicine was prescribed?
- What can I expect it to do?
- How will I know if it's working?
- When and how should I take it?
- When should I *not* take it?
- Could it produce any side effects?
- Is it all right to drive while I'm taking this medicine?
- Can I take it with others I may need?
- Are there any foods or beverages I should avoid?
- How long do I need to take this medicine?
- When will I need another doctor's appointment?

In other words, if you don't know *all* about the drug you're prescribed for pain, *ask.* Or look it up. Good sources of information include the *Physicians' Desk Reference* and *About Your Medicines,* both of which should be available at your local library.

Source Notes

Chapter 1

Pages 8-9

"How Pains Compare" adapted from *Conquering Pain* by Dr. Sampson Lipton. Copyright 1984 by Sampson Lipton. Reprinted by permission of the publisher, Prentice-Hall, Inc., Englewood Cliffs, N.J.

Chapter 2

Page 13

"Specialists in Relief" statistics adapted from *Back-Ache Relief* by Arthur C. Klein and Dava Sobel (New York: Random House, 1985).

Page 16

"Test Your Back" adapted from *Goodbye Backache* by David Imrie, M.D. (New York: Arco, 1983).

Chapter 4

Page 39

"Exercise against Arthritis" adapted from *The Arthritis Helpbook* by Kate Lorig and James Fries, pages 28, 31, 33, 35, 38, 41, 44. Copyright 1980 by Addison-Wesley, Reading, Massachusetts; reprinted with permission.

Pages 42-43

"Help Yourself to Less Pain" adapted from "Self-Help Manual for Patients with Arthritis" by the Arthritis Health Professions Section of the Arthritis Foundation.

Chapter 5

Page 69

Information on shingles treatment originally cited in "Herpes Zoster: The Treatment and Prevention of Neuralgia with Adenosine Monophosphate," by S. Harvey Sklar et al., *Journal of the American Medical Association*, vol. 253, no. 10, March 8, 1985.

Chapter 7

Page 93

"Measuring Your Pain" adapted from "The McGill Pain Questionnaire: Major Properties and Scoring Methods," by Ronald Melzack, *Pain*, 1975.

Chapter 8

Pages 108-109

"How to Give a Foot Massage" adapted from *The Massage Book* by George Downing (New York: Random House—the Bookworks, 1972).

Chapter 9

Page 125

"Hypnosis Quiz" adapted from "The Medically Tested Bad-Habit Breaker" by Barbara DeBetz, M.D., and Stephanie Brush, *Self*, June 1981. Reprinted by permission of the authors.

Chapter 12

Page 156

"When to See a Doctor for Pain" adapted from *The American Medical Association Family Medical Guide*, edited by Jeffrey R. N. Kunz, M.D. (New York: Random House, 1982).

Photography Credits

Cover: Angelo M. Caggiano.
Staff Photographers— Angelo M. Caggiano: pp. 10-11; 52-53; 54; 78; 90-91; 103; 130-131; 142-149. Isabelle Delmotte: p. 123. Carl Doney: pp. 24-25; 127; 141; 150-151. T. L. Gettings: p. 116. Donna Hornberger: pp. 5; 15; 21; 27; 30; 32; 33; 41; 42-43; 51; 56; 61; 65; 76; 83; 85; 89; 97; 107; 115; 118-119; 121; 129; 135; 139; 155; 161. Mark Lenny: p. 113. Andrea Mihalik: p. 39, top left. Alison Miksch: pp. 27, b/w; 74; 106; 115, b/w; 128; 129, b/w; 132; 161, b/w. Paul Pelak: pp. 16-17; 18; 23; 29; 39, bottom left, top center and bottom center, top right and bottom right; 67; 71; 108-109. Margaret Skrovanek: pp. 34; 47; 72-73; 110-111; 153. Christie C. Tito: pp. 3, left; 79. Sally Shenk Ullman: pp. 36-37.

Other Photographers— Herb Ball: p. 21. Cicciro Donnely: pp. viii-1. Kurt Foss: pp. 139, b/w; 155, b/w. Barbara Fritz: pp. 104-105. Elliott Kaufman: p. 59. Tony Korody/ Sygma: p. 57. Mike McGrath: pp. 41, b/w; 51, b/w. Ellen Michaud: p. 65, b/w. John M. Roberts: p. 64.

Additional Photographs Courtesy of— The Bettman Archive, Inc.: pp. 98; 159. Devaney Stock Photos: pp. 3, right; 101. Ralph Lester: p. 135, b/w. The Miami Dolphins: p. 89, b/w. NASA: p. 19. Photo Researchers, Inc.: p. 3, center. Rodale Press Photography Department: pp. 86; 127. Richard Ruth Satz: p. 82. Smithsonian Institution: p. 120. Joan Throckmorton: p. 15, b/w. The Union-Tribune Publishing Co.: p. 136.

Photographic Styling Credits

Renee R. Keith: pp. 18; 23; 29; 67. Kay Seng Lichthardt: p. 74. Debra Minotti: pp. 18; 23; 39; 54; 56; 71; 78; 90-91; 108-109. Kurt Swinehart: pp. 54; 103; 110-111. J. C. Vera: pp. 72-73. Mary Ellen Whitaker: pp. 42-43.

Illustration Credits

Bascove: pp. 2; 26; 102. Susan Blubaugh: pp. 12; 84. Mellisa Edmonds: pp. 8-9; 54. Susan Gray: pp. 20; 157. John Knutila: pp. 116-117, sculpture. Elwood Smith: pp. 66; 77. Wendy Wray: p. 49.

Special Thanks to— Allen Organ Sales, Macungie, Pa.; Bickel's Surgical Supply, Bethlehem, Pa.; Kahle's Music Store, Emmaus, Pa.; the patients and staff of the pain clinic at the University of Washington, Seattle, Wash.

Index

Rodale Press, Inc., publishes PREVENTION®, the better health magazine.
For information on how to order your subscription,
write to PREVENTION®, Emmaus, PA 18049.